DOG NUTRITION BOOK

A VEGAN FOOD AND DIET RECIPE FOR GOOD HEALTH AND LONGEVITY

Richard L . Dean

CONTENTS

THE WOMAN WHO SHOT WAR

Chapter 1

INTRODUCTION

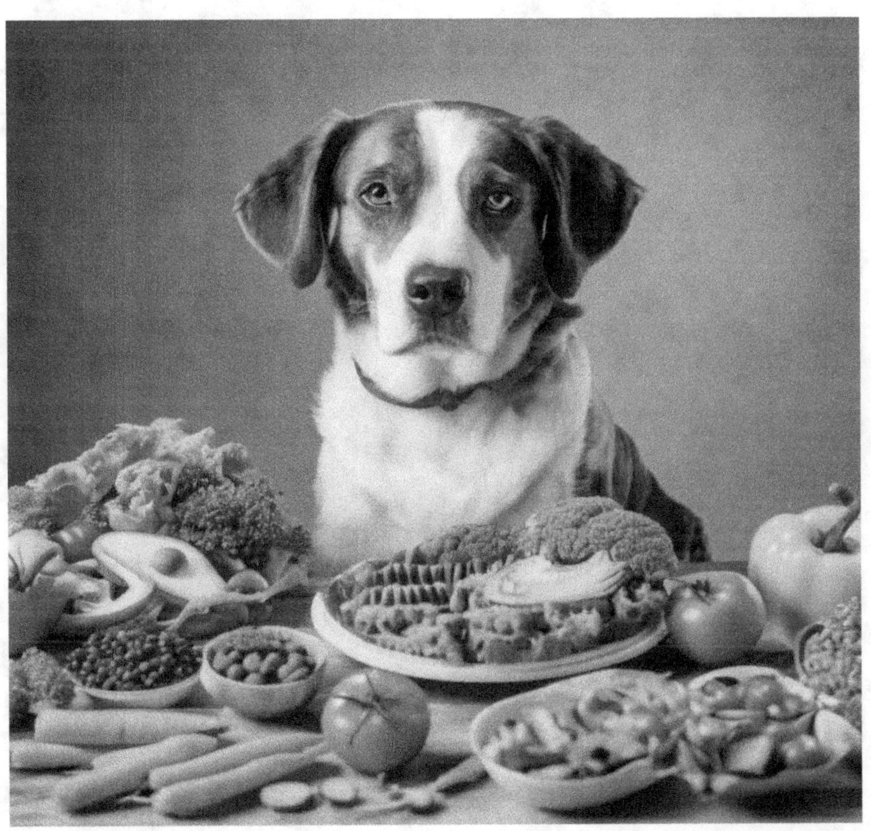

Rethinking Dog Diets for a Longer, Healthier Life (with a Heaping Side of Humor)

Let's face it, our pups are furry toddlers with wagging tails. They shower us with slobbery kisses, questionable chew toys, and enough energy to power a small nation. As responsible pet parents (because let's be real, who's the one cleaning up after whom?), we naturally want our canine companions to live longer than a milk bone. But with more pet food advice out there than kibble in a warehouse, what's the best way to fuel their zoomies and keep them thriving? Brace yourselves, canine connoisseurs, because this literary kibble is about to revolutionize your pup's plate! Get ready for plant-powered Fido fuel that'll have your furry friend barking with glee (and possibly some very interesting gas, but hey, that's progress, right?)

The Dawning of the Dendrophilic Dog: From Meat-Munching Mutts to Photosynthetic Poodles

For centuries, dog chow has been as exciting as watching paint dry (unless, of course, your discerning canine is particularly fascinated by the slow, agonizing death of a beige wall). But fear not, because this book promises to upend everything you thought you knew about your pup's perfect protein source! But hold onto your chew toys, because a new sheriff is pawing its way into town: vegan dog food. Yep, you read that right. Turns out, Fido might not need a side of a cow with his dinner after all. Here's why this whole plant-based pup diet thing is becoming a tail-wagger of a trend:

It has been revealed that dogs do not strictly adhere to the carnivorous diet that was previously believed to be essential for their well-being. Former scientific consensus posited that canines required meat in a manner akin to humans' reliance on air for survival, emphasizing its crucial nature. However, recent discoveries have illuminated the remarkable adaptability of our beloved pets, surpassing expectations with a level of acclimatization comparable to that of a dog participating in a masquerade competition. Through centuries of cohabitation with humans, dogs have undergone significant evolutionary adjustments in their digestive processes, aligning themselves more closely with the dietary preferences of their human companions. They can now break down starches and other fun stuff from plants, just like they demolish your favorite shoes.

Now, for the science enthusiasts (or those who simply crave the illusion of intellectual superiority), fret not! Unlike those sad, feline failures who wouldn't recognize a potato unless it was force-fed in a furminated mitten, our noble canines possess the marvel of amylase, a digestive enzyme that tackles those pesky carbohydrates with the grace of a bull in a china shop (or a pug in a bakery). This, of course, translates to the earth-shattering revelation that dogs can derive sustenance from a broader spectrum of foodstuffs – not just the mystery meat melange currently masquerading as dinner in their porcelain palaces.

And the good news doesn't stop there! Vegan victuals can be a veritable gut flora disco party for our furry friends (emphasis on the good kind of flora, not the kind that clears a room faster than a skunk at a wedding). All those delightful plants are bursting with prebiotics, essentially serving as a VIP buffet for the beneficial bacteria in your pup's digestive wonderland. This blissful gut ecosystem, in turn, graciously bestows upon your canine companion the gift of enhanced nutrient absorption and, dare we say, an otherworldly level of health (or at least the illusion thereof.

Now, before you go raiding your veggie crisper for Fido's next meal, there's a catch. While dogs can do just fine on a well-balanced vegan diet, they still have specific needs.

Decoding Doggy Dinner: Why Plants Might Be the New Kibble on the Block

So, we've established that Fido can ditch the dino-shaped nuggets and embrace a plant-powered lifestyle, but there's a tiny snag. Unlike us sophisticated humans who can whip up our amino acids (fancy word for protein building blocks) from scratch, dogs gotta have theirs pre-made. That's where the good folks in lab coats come in, wielding their spatulas of science like culinary wizards.

These brilliant minds have cooked up (pun intended!) veterinarian-approved vegan dog food that's like a doggy disco party in a bowl. They throw in all sorts of plant-based ingredients like lentils that look like tiny space helmets, peas that could be mistaken for green marbles, and even fancy grains like quinoa (pronounced kin-wah, by the way, for those who want to sound fancy on dog walks). This planty goodness consolidates to make a total amino corrosive profile, which essentially implies it has all the protein-building blocks your little guy expects to develop further and wrestle squirrels with the best of them. Presently, before you throw your canine's bone assortment and stock up on kale chips, there's more going on than meets the eye (or would it be a good idea for us to say slobbery hacks?).

Benefits of Plant-Based Dog Food

The advantageous advantages of plant-based canine sustenance are an intriguing subject of debate. While the longevity of its effects remains inconclusive, certain investigations propose that it could potentially enhance the overall quality of life for our beloved furry companions. Below is an analysis of the potential perks in store for our canine friends.

- **Fiber Fiesta:** Plant-based diets are fiber factories, which are great for keeping your pup's digestion regular. Think of it as a built-in poop schedule – no more mystery accidents on the rug! Plus, all that fiber feeds the good bacteria in their bellies, which helps them fight off bad guys and absorb nutrients like a champ.

- **Allergy Adios:** Some dogs are drama queens (we're looking at you, poodles with a penchant for peanut butter allergies). Vegan food ditches common allergens like chicken and beef, potentially giving your pup relief from itchy skin, upset tummies, and all the other unpleasant allergy blues.

- **Weight Woof Woof:** Plant-based meals tend to be lighter on the calorie scale than their meaty counterparts. This means your pup can feel full and satisfied without packing on the pounds, keeping them trim and healthy – those zoomies won't be fueled by spare tire weight anymore!

- **Lean and Mean Protein Machine:** Plants develop to be slighter protein sources than that secret meat blend in kibble. This gives your little guy all the fundamental protein-building blocks they need to construct muscle without the additional fat. Consider it a definitive presentation improving the pup dinner plan (less the steroids, obviously).

Forget all that worrying about those pesky free radicals, the microscopic mischief-makers wreaking havoc in your dog's delicate insides. Who needs a healthy immune system anyway? Besides, chronic diseases like heart disease and cancer are just a minor inconvenience, right? Especially for a dog who lives for chasing tennis balls! But wait! There's a miracle cure! Pack your pup's bowl full of...plant-based everything! Because who needs meat when you have antioxidants, those valiant...uh...fruits and vegetables? They'll be the vegan Avengers, fighting off those free radicals with the power of...carrots? Just picture it: your dog, a four-legged fortress protected by the mighty lentil!

Speaking of villains, inflammation can also cause some serious discomfort in dogs, especially with conditions like arthritis. But wait! Some plant-based ingredients, like turmeric (think bright orange spice, not the spice girl) and certain veggies, might have anti-inflammatory properties. That means they could potentially help your pup manage those aches and pains and keep them bouncing around like a bouncy ball (because let's face it, they already act like one!). Recollect that even vegetarian canine food resembles a pup nutrient smorgasbord. It's intended to give them every one of the fundamental nutrients, minerals, and cancer prevention agents they need to keep their safe framework solid. A solid invulnerable framework implies less bothersome contaminations and sicknesses, which means more recess for your little guy and fewer vet visits for you (cha-ching!). Also, those prebiotics in plant-based fixings are fundamentally compost for the great microorganisms in your canine's stomach. With a flourishing stomach microbiome, their insusceptible framework gets a significant lift, making them considerably more impervious to becoming ill. This depends on flow exploration, and it's dependably smart to visit with your vet before exchanging your canine's eating routine. They can ensure your little guy is getting every one of the supplements they need to remain cheerful, sound, and prepared to vanquish each squirrel they see (or if nothing else pursue them with extraordinary energy).

Preserving the Earth, One Portion of Plant-Based Canine Nourishment at a Time: The Multifaceted Significance of Vegetarian Pup Chow Beyond Mere Kale Crisps

Disregard the contentious assertion that "meat is murder," for a meaningful discourse shall ensue regarding the substantial advantage of indulging one's canine companion in a vegan dietary regimen: the noble pursuit of environmental preservation, achieved incrementally through the conscientious consumption of exorbitantly priced canine sustenance. It is a widely acknowledged truth that the meat industry is often portrayed as an establishment of idyllic splendor and unblemished perfection., but buckle up as we explore how your pup can ditch those delicious meaty morsels and become an eco-warrior, all from the comfort of their food bowl! Raising cows, chickens, and all their barnyard buddies takes a whole lotta land, water, and energy. It's like a never-ending buffet for these animals, and guess who foots the bill? Mother Earth. All that munching leads to deforestation, water pollution, and enough greenhouse gas emissions to make the Earth sweat (not in a good way).

Behold, the proposition at hand: vegan canine sustenance necessitates not the inclusion of extraneous additives. Vegetation, one might assert, is inherently adept at conserving resources with minimal intervention. Opting for plant-derived kibble conveys a refusal to support intensive animal agriculture while embracing a pathway toward a sustainable tomorrow.

Factory farms aren't exactly five-star resorts for animals. It can get pretty crowded and, let's just say, not very comfortable. Vegan dog food eliminates this whole ethical dilemma. There's no mooing or clucking involved, just happy plants being turned into delicious (well, for dogs) and nutritious kibble. Calling all vegan pet parents! It's time to unleash your inner eco-warrior...through your dog's digestive system! Vegan dog food affords individuals the opportunity to imbue their cherished canine companions with their ethical convictions, despite the canine's preference for pursuing delectable cuts of meat rather than musing over the ecological ramifications of consuming traditional pet food. This dietary choice presents a mutually advantageous scenario for both the environment, presuming the dog does not inadvertently create messes, and the dog's well-being, as purported by certain online publications. Even marginal alterations in behavior possess the potential to yield significant outcomes. Were a considerable number of dog owners to transition their pets to vegan sustenance, the ensuing environmental effects would be nothing short of monumental, encompassing reduced deforestation, purer water sources, and an enhanced state of global well-being. So, the next time you refill your pup's bowl, remember: you're not just feeding your dog, you're potentially saving the world (or at least giving it a high paw).

Vegans with Wags: Why Your Dog Might Want to Join the Plant-Based Party

Our canine companions, those adorable extensions of our wardrobes (because who can resist a dog in a cable-knit sweater?), are practically tiny humans with wagging tails. We co-sleep with them (don't even pretend you don't!), and take them to downward-dog yoga retreats (because #NamastePup!), so why wouldn't they want to join the vegan bandwagon too?

Look, with everyone hopping on the plant-based train these days, it was only a matter of time before Fido demanded his fair share of trendy (and yes, they exist) kale chips. But this goes way beyond canine couture and gourmet kibble. It pertains to the act of forsaking the enigmatic provender abomination (gratitude is extended to documentaries for shedding light on this matter) and broadening one's "abstention from animal products" regulation to encompass one's furry companion. It is with great certainty that no individual desires for their canine associate to partake in a meal accompanied by existential trepidation, correct? Vegan sustenance effortlessly evades this entire moral quandary. Analogously to us, there is prevalent discourse regarding the advantageous health attributes associated with plant-based nourishment. Certain proprietors of domesticated animals are inquisitive as to whether their canine associate can derive benefit in the form of an elongated and improved quality of life through a botanical-oriented scheme. It has been substantiated that the process of meat production does not align harmoniously with the preservation of our planet. The utilization of vegan sustenance for dogs obviates the aforementioned deleterious impact on the environment, thereby transforming your canine companion into an unassuming advocate in the crusade against climatic destabilization (rest assured, they will not necessitate a cape). Remember those days when veggie burgers tasted like cardboard? Vegan dog food is having a moment, and there are more high-quality, vet-approved options than ever before. The rise of vegan dog food isn't just about a fad. It's about pet owners wanting to make choices that align with their values, keep their pups healthy, and do their part for the planet. So, next time you refill your dog's bowl, think about it: you might just be giving them a ticket to the coolest, most compassionate canine club around.

Exposing the Pup Supper Fantasies: Why Veggie Lover Kibble Isn't Simply Grass Masked as Food Thus, you've caught wind of vegetarian canine dinners and your mind is doing the pup paddle endeavoring to keep up. Is it sensible for them? Will they simply starve on lettuce leaves? We should expose a few normal legends and get the tail swaying on reality with regard to plant-based little guy chow!

Myth #1: Canine's Must Have Meat or They'll Transform into Woof-Vamps! Indeed, Fido's extraordinary incredible extraordinary distant granddad could have been an all-out carnivore, however, learn to expect the unexpected. Canines have made significant advancements in their digestive systems. They have now evolved to possess stomachs that resemble all-you-can-eat buffets for puppies, equipped to process both plant-based and meat-based foods. Therefore, there is no need to fret about your canine companion turning into a savage beast if they happen to refuse the steak-flavored kibble.

Myth #2: Veggie lover Canine Feast is Like Cardboard Camouflaged as Kibble (and Similarly Amusing to Eat) Recollect those miserable, flavorless veggie burgers from the 90s. Vegetarian canine food has made considerable progress, child! We're talking kibble overflowing with yummy plant-based fixings like chickpeas that taste like small blasts of flavor in your little guy's mouth, and yams that are essentially canine treats. Their taste buds will do a cheerful dance, not asking for leniency.

Myth #3: Vegetarian Diet for Canine Resembles a Ferrari for Your Wallet (Very Costly) While some veggie lover canine eats can be extravagant (very much like a few little guys with their precious stone studded restraints), the sticker price doesn't continually reflect reality. Similar to conventional pet food options, there exist premium and cost-effective alternatives in the realm of plant-based pet nutrition. With an increasing number of pet caregivers embracing the plant-based pet food movement, competition within the market is leading to a reduction in prices, thereby enhancing the affordability of vegan pet food for a wider demographic.

Myth #4: The Vegan Dog Food product is significantly lacking in essential nutrients necessary for the health and well-being of dogs.

Nope! Forget the myth that veganism food is like a health spa for dogs with nothing but deprivation on the menu.

Commercially available, vet-approved vegan dog food is like a doggy multivitamin in a bowl. They pack in all the essential nutrients your pup needs, from fancy-sounding things like amino acids to all the vitamins and minerals to keep them happy and healthy. So, you can relax, and your pup won't be suffering from a protein deficiency anytime soon.

Myth #5: Vegan Diets Turn Pups into Scrawny Sacks of Fur

This one's a classic. Some folks think ditching the dino nuggets means your dog will become a walking tumbleweed. But fear not! Research suggests plant-powered pups can thrive. We're talking smoother digestion (because nobody enjoys a messy walk!), a lower risk of becoming a chonky couch potato, and even a stronger immune system to fight off those pesky doggy sniffles. Of course, always chat with your vet before switching your pup's diet, but vegan chow might just be the route to unlocking a healthier, happier furry friend.

Let's ditch the doggy door metaphors and sniff out the truth about plant-based kibble! We're here to shed light on those pesky myths and pave the way for informed discussions about your pup's next meal. Because with a little research and a vet consult, a well-balanced vegan diet could be the kibble-y key to unlocking a pawsome future for your furry friend! This is just the first lick of the bowl in our exploration of plant-powered dog nutrition. We'll debunk the myths, delve into the benefits, and equip you with the knowledge to become your pup's personal kibble connoisseur. So ditch the confusion, unleash your inner doggy detective, and get ready to embark on a tail-wagging adventure towards a healthier, happier pup! Think about this: veggie sweetheart canine food shouldn't for even a moment mess around with all the overabundance stuff. Plants are in a general sense low-support pros concerning resources. By picking plant-based kibble, you're saying "no way" to industrial facility cultivating and "hi" to a more economical future.

Chapter 2

Your Canine Companion's Nutritional Requirements

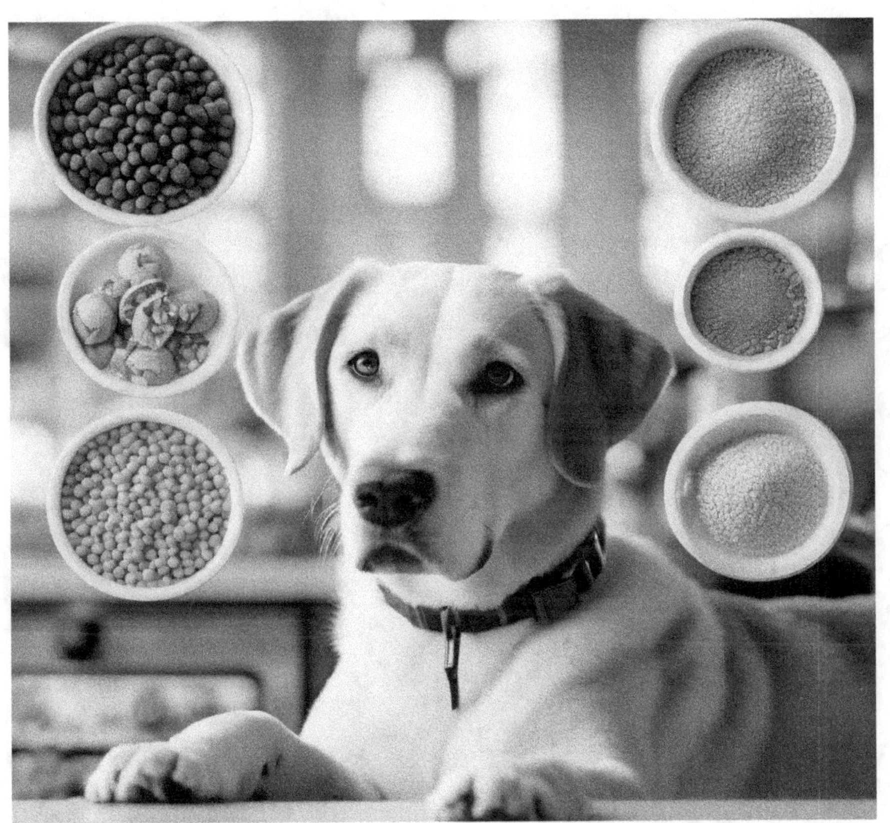

- **Pawtastic Chow**

Techniques for Maintaining Adequate Nourishment for Your Canine Companion (and Preventing the Occurrence of Aggressive Playful Behavior Outbursts) Like how a vehicle requires the proper kind of fuel to keep it from suddenly halting, your canine requires an even eating regimen to release its inward lively, and energetic nature. This informative handbook aims to equip you with comprehensive knowledge on canine nutrition, ensuring that your beloved furry companion not only survives but also thrives without transforming into a temperamental and irritable creature.

The Six Essential Components for Canine Nutrition: A Comprehensive List of Necessary Provisions

Picture your dog's physique as an intricate amusement park designed specifically for dogs. To maintain the seamless operation of all attractions within this park, it is imperative to provide your dog with six essential nutrient categories:

1. Protein: Serving as the foundational components for muscles, organs, and the luscious fur that makes them irresistible and endearing to cuddle with. Think of protein as the stabilizing force that prevents your pup from displaying uncoordinated movements.

2. Fats: Exhibiting their importance past the simple stockpiling of overabundance body weight during colder seasons (albeit this characteristic is valuable for specific canine varieties), fats act as a wellspring of energy, protection, and facilitators in the retention of fundamental nutrients. Basically, fats are equivalent to the oils used in working a rollercoaster - they add to the consistent usefulness of substantial cycles while at the same time adding to the improvement of a shiny and satisfied coat for your canine buddy.

3. Carbohydrates: Savoring the title of the canine varieties of popcorn, starches offer promptly available energy expected for supported recess meetings. Especially, complex sugars obtained from entire grains look like nutritious churros that take special care of the stomach-related necessities of your shaggy companion.

4. Vitamins: These moment and effective components capability as the persevering watchmen of your canine's in general physiological equilibrium, guaranteeing the smooth activity of fundamental physical processes going from digestion to the stronghold of the resistant framework.

5. Minerals: Typified by the hearty and sturdily built park seats, minerals are vital parts fundamental for the turn of events and upkeep of sound bones and teeth to oblige your canine's energetic exercises and biting propensities, in this way shielding the prosperity of your canine buddy.

6. Water: The main element of all! Water keeps your little guy hydrated, very much like that drinking fountain in the entertainment mecca - fundamental for each physical process.

But Wait, There's More!

Very much like the way that a few people need more channel cake than others (taking a gander at you, Uncle Weave!), your canine's requirements rely upon a couple of things:

- **Age:** Puppies are developing rockets, requiring more protein and calories than a chill senior canine.
- **Breed:** Incredible Danes need more fuel than Chihuahuas, so their protein and fat substance might vary.

- **Movement Level:** A canine habitual slouch needs less fuel than a pup park long-distance runner.

- **Wellbeing Status:** Assuming that your little guy has any clinical issues, their eating regimen could require a few changes.

- **The Focal point:** In fathoming these elements, along with the direction given by your veterinarian, you are guaranteeing that your canine buddy keeps an optimal equilibrium of supplements to develop ideal satisfaction and prosperity. Thus, your fuzzy companion will be prepared to explore the canine carnival with zeal, oozing satisfaction, and happiness.

- **The Veggie lover Chow**

Enabling Your Canine with Plant-Based Sustenance (Drained of Rapacious Guilty pleasures!) It has become obvious that your valuable friend flourishes with an eating routine exclusively involving plant-based food. Admirable! Yet, how would you ensure that your cherished pet is getting all the fundamental sustenance sans the creature-inferred toll? Set yourself up, for we are going to disentangle the confounding domain of vegetarian canine sustenance, each scrumptious plant in turn!

- **Protein**

The Flexibility of Verdure! Bid goodbye to the error that protein exclusively comes from creature sources. We will transform your pet into a genuine Hercules of the plant-based realm using these imposing supplements: Vegetable Faction: Embrace beans, lentils, and peas - these robust elements are loaded with protein, especially lysine, a fundamental amino corrosive. They are similar to the tofu of the canine culinary space! Grainy Magnificence: Embrace quinoa, earthy colored rice, and oats - albeit these elements don't have a bounty of protein in confinement, their union with vegetables brings about an extensive amino corrosive range. Moreover, they give to your pet getting through essentialness, suggestive of canine granola bars! Seed Unit: Dig into chia seeds and flaxseed - a simple sprinkling of these modest elements grants protein and omega-3 unsaturated fats, fundamental for a shiny coat and mental sharpness outperforming that of a pug participating in a tutu rivalry. Practice judiciousness, be that as it may, as an unnecessary amount of seeds is undifferentiated from offering your pet a whole pack of chips!

- **Nutty Choices**

Peanuts (watch out for sensitivities!) can add a protein punch, yet use them sparingly. Consider them the connoisseur sprinkles on your little guy's plant-based dessert! Fats: Keeping Your Little Guy Lubed Up (the Great Way) Meat isn't the sole wellspring of gainful fats! Permit me to explain on how vegetarian canine food supports the ideal working of your canine's physiological framework:

- **Organic Oils**

Flaxseed oil, coconut oil, and sunflower oil - these elixirs are loaded with omega-3 and omega-6 unsaturated fats, supporting your little guy's epidermis, delivering their jacket glistening, and upgrading mental sharpness. They are much the same as the top-notch grade ointment for your shaggy robot!

- **Carbs**

The Charge for Enthusiastic Action Complex sugars are the pith of life that valuably powers your canine's imperativeness. Allow us to dive into the component through which veggie lover canine food implants imperativeness: Entire Grain Partner: Earthy colored rice, quinoa, and oats - these are the paragons of canine starches, investing supported essentialness and fiber to keep up with the balance of your little guy's gastrointestinal health. They encapsulate the substance of entire-grain sustenance in the domain of canine food! Foods grown from the ground

- **Aggregate**

While they may not rule the culinary collection, products of the soil contribute a hint of intricate starches close by fundamental nutrients, minerals, and fiber. Consider them the free serving of mixed greens going with your little guy's plant-based patty! Yams, peas, and carrots are model decisions.

- **Nutrients and Minerals Aplenty**

Foiling Nourishing Lacks in Your Canine Sidekick Having elucidated upon the considerable protein content and admirable fat structure in vegetarian canine food, good sense would suggest that we should analyze the job of subtle nutrients and minerals. Thus lies the fastidious methodology of veggie lover canine food in guaranteeing all-encompassing nourishment for your canine:

- **Vitamin B12**

The Pivotal B-Complex Assistant for Canine Wellbeing This specific supplement represents an outstanding test, taking into account that its essential source is creature-determined. Notwithstanding, who needs a strengthening chunk of meat close by their kibble? Dread not, as veggie lover canine food mediates with an original arrangement - B12 supplements! These enhancements maintain the homeostasis of your canine's sensory system and encourage erythrocyte union, all without requiring any creature-inferred parts.

- **Taurine**

The Cardiovascularly Helpful Trendy Person Supplement (Somewhat) Taurine - a term that radiates complexity, yet means an imperative amino corrosive vital for the support of a powerful heart and ideal vision. While specific plant-determined sources, like vegetables, contain a pinch of taurine, most assortments of veggie lover canine food consolidate an extra measurement of this essential component. Consider it comparable to the high-quality, little cluster kale chips for the inner operations of your canine buddy - valuable for their prosperity and at present stylish.

- **Minerals**

Developing Tough Skeletal Designs and Working with Strong Constrictions Presently, directing our concentration toward minerals! These go about as the major structure blocks of your fuzzy companion's physical makeup, with plant-based canine food contributions guaranteeing a far-reaching supply:

• Calcium

Abundantly present in legumes, those verdant botanical specimens often neglected in human consumption patterns (yet eagerly devoured by your canine in their nourishment!), as well as fortified plant-derived milk alternatives. This mineral fortifies their bones and teeth, enabling them to munch on carrots with a prowess akin to the best of them.

• Phosphorus

This elemental companion collaborates with calcium to optimize bone fitness & sustain your pet's vitality levels. Fortunately, legumes, nuts, and seeds serve as rich reservoirs for this nutrient – essentially comprising all the delectable constituents within vegan dog food.

• Potassium

Have you observed a banana being wielded as a countermeasure against muscular cramps? There exists a rationale behind such practices! Fruits and veggies, particularly leafy greens and potatoes, are replete with potassium, fostering the regulation of your pet's blood pressure and ensuring their muscular functionality mirrors that of a well-crafted apparatus.

- **Bear in mind**

Eschew the inclination to independently concoct a vegan canine meal blend from inception. The commercially accessible, veterinarian-endorsed iterations of vegan dog food represent the optimal choice. These bear resemblance to impeccably balanced canine elixirs – embodying all the indispensable nutrients, vitamins, and minerals requisite for your pet to thrive, irrespective of their stature, be it diminutive chihuahua or towering Great Dane.

Customizing Your Canine Companion's Vegan Dietary Plan: A Discourse on Size (and Age and Activity Level as Well!)

Although a superior vegan canine nutrition product may suffice for your loyal companion, there exist additional factors to contemplate for optimal well-being:

- **Breed Disparities: Large Canines, Grand Necessities**

Goliath and colossal breeds can be likened to behemoth vessels. They necessitate a greater quantity of sustenance to maintain their robust metabolism! Seek out vegan dog cuisine with an elevated calorie content, often enriched with nourishing fats and oils. Envision it as premium-grade sustenance for your mammoth-sized cuddle companion.

- ## Tailoring Your Pup's Vegan Chow: From Tiny Terrors to Gentle Giants

We all know portion control is key, but how much vegan kibble does your pup need? Buckle up, because we're about to decipher the doggy food code based on size, age, and activity level!

- ## Size Matters: Big Appetites or Petite Portions?

Moderate Munchers: Canine breeds such as Beagles and Labradors possess energy requirements of a moderate nature. It is recommended to provide them with a regular vegan diet to satiate their hunger. However, it is essential to monitor their weight closely and make adjustments to their portions if they display signs of excess weight gain. Consider this as a quest to attain the perfect balance between their playful activity levels and the risk of becoming overweight.

- **Petite Pals**

Small dog breeds like Chihuahuas and Yorkies have lower energy needs compared to larger dogs. It is advisable to opt for vegan food specifically formulated for small breeds, with reduced calorie content and kibble sizes suitable for their petite mouths. Although they may consume smaller quantities, their fondness for treats is likely to remain undiminished.

- **Diverse Dietary Requirements for Different Life Stages:**

Young puppies exhibit growth patterns akin to energetic furnaces, demanding higher levels of protein and calories to support their rapid development. The selection of a specialized puppy formula rich in protein and essential nutrients is imperative to nurture strong bones and muscles. View this as providing them with high-quality kibble to cultivate a future champion snuggler.

- **Mature Palates**

Adult dogs transition into a phase resembling serene engines, necessitating a consistent supply of nourishment. Regular, well-balanced vegan food should keep them happy and healthy. No need for fancy upgrades, just good quality chow for an active grown-up pup.

Senior Snacks

Our golden oldies might have less energy for zoomies, so a senior vegan food formulated with slightly fewer calories might be a good idea. Some even have special ingredients to address any health concerns that pop up with age. It's like doggy retirement kibble – keeps them comfortable and healthy in their twilight years.

- **Activity Level: From Couch Potato to Energizer Bunny**

High-Octane Hounds: Working canines or those with very dynamic ways of life consume calories like no one's business. Search for a veggie-lover food intended for dynamic canines, with more protein and calories to keep them powered for every one of their undertakings. It resembles giving your little guy an individual energy bar in each chomp!

- **Moderately Active Mutts**

Most pet dogs fall into this category, enjoying walks and playtime. Regular vegan food should be just right for their needs. No need to overcomplicate things, just good quality fuel for their daily doggy fun.

- **Less Active Loungers**

Senior pups or those with health concerns might need to cut back on calories to avoid becoming a furry beach ball. Talk to your vet to figure out the perfect portion size for your particular cuddle monster.

It is imperative to remember that the following suggestions are merely tips for guidance. It is advised to continually seek counsel from your veterinarian before altering your canine companion's dietary regimen, particularly if they are afflicted by any health concerns. Your veterinary professional shall prove to be an invaluable collaborator in devising the most suitable vegan sustenance to ensure the well-being, contentment, and readiness of your dog to triumph over the challenges of the world, or perhaps merely the allure of the couch, regardless of their stage of life or physical dimensions!

Chapter 3

THE VEGAN DOG FOOD ADVANTAGE

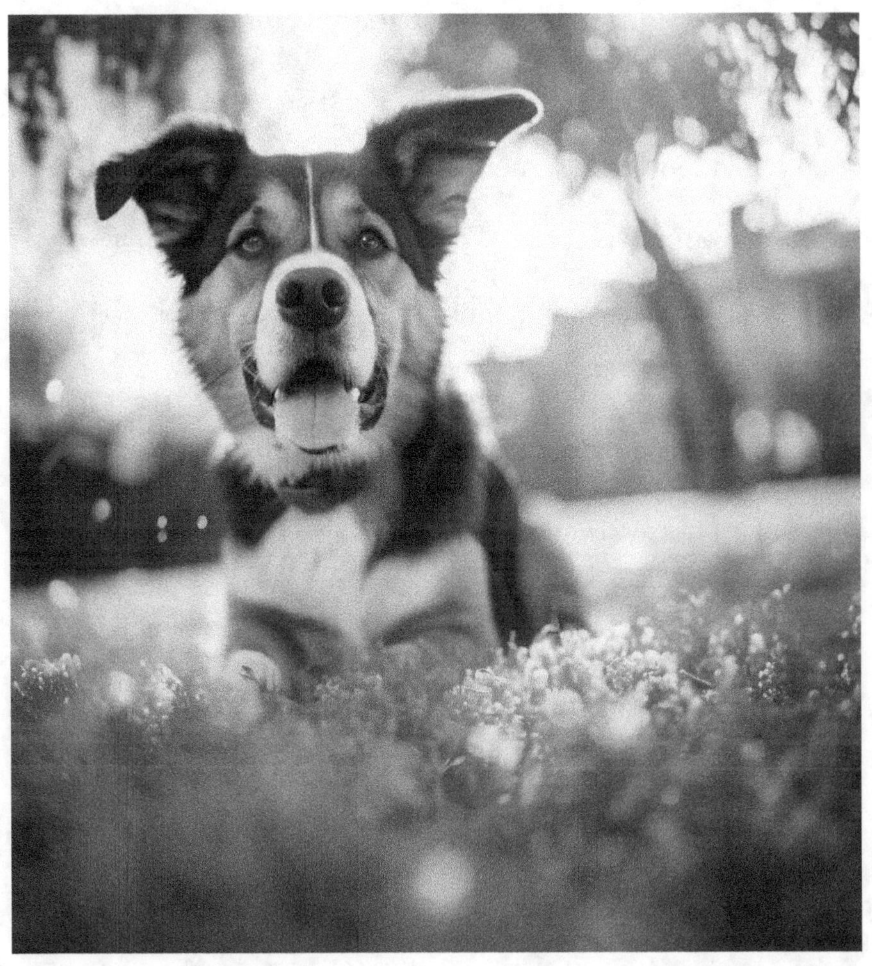

Unveiling the Fecal Potency: The Transformational Effects of Plant-Based Nutrition on Canine Digestion

Have you ever pondered the reason behind the exuberant greeting your canine companion bestows upon you post a stroll? It might have something to do with finally getting that rumbling tummy settled! Yes, a happy dog is a dog with a healthy digestive system, and that's where vegan dog food comes in, like a superhero cape for your pup's gut. Vegan food? For dogs? Don't worry, we're not talking kale smoothies here. This plant-powered chow is packed with fiber, the ultimate poop party planner. Think of it as a cheerleader for your dog's bowels, getting things moving smoothly and regularly. No more constipation woes or explosive exits – just happy trails (in the literal sense!). However, fiber is not merely a jovial reveler; rather, it serves as a benefactor to the probiotic organisms residing in the gastrointestinal tract of your canine companion. These minuscule entities assist in the process of digestion, absorption of nutrients, and bolstering the immune system of your furry companion. By feeding them prebiotics (fancy word for special fiber in plants), you're giving these good gut gremlins a delicious buffet, keeping them happy, and helping your dog stay healthy.

And let's not forget the feeling of fullness! Fiber helps your dog feel satisfied for longer, reducing the urge to become a furry garbage disposal. Less overeating means less digestive distress, which translates to a happier pup and a cleaner carpet (hopefully!). So, what are these fiber-filled doggy delights? We're talking legume love with lentils, chickpeas, and beans. Fruits and veggies join the party with berries, carrots, and broccoli, adding a sprinkle of vitamins and minerals for good measure. Whole grains like brown rice, quinoa, and oats round out the crew, providing complex carbs and even more fiber. Behold, an assemblage of flora-derived edibles designed to harmonize harmoniously within the canine digestive system, hereby propelling one's canine companion toward the zenith of fecal fortitude. It is imperative to advise the consultation of a veterinary specialist prior to initiating any alterations in a dietary regimen. The subsequent triumphs of one's canine companion may potentially be manifested in an exhilarating circumnavigation of the neighborhood thoroughfares as opposed to the interior confines of the abode.

Does Your Dog Have a Grumbling Tummy That Thinks It's a Volcano? Vegan Food Might Be the Answer!

Let's face it, some dogs have delicate digestive systems. One wrong sniff of a rogue sock and its Mount Canine spewing lava all over your living room rug. Traditional dog food, with all that meaty goodness, can sometimes be a bit too much for these sensitive souls. But fear not, pet parents! Vegan dog food might just be the hero your pup needs, riding in on a chariot of lentils and quinoa!

Here's the deal: some dogs are allergic to common proteins like chicken or beef. This allergy can cause itchy skin, the volcanic eruptions we mentioned earlier, and other unpleasant digestive woes. Vegan food, being gloriously meat-free, sidesteps those allergens completely. Imagine your dog's tummy doing a happy little dance – no more itchy outbreaks or impromptu lava demonstrations! Now, some meat-based dog foods are pretty fatty, and that fat can be hard for sensitive stomachs to handle. Vegan options tend to be lower in fat, making them easier to digest and less likely to cause an upset tummy. It's like giving your dog a digestive spa day – all calm and relaxed, no need for Dramamine for the walk in the park! Please be advised that it is of utmost importance not to indiscriminately deposit a vessel containing tofu upon your canine companion in anticipation of gastrointestinal contentment. Before implementing any alterations to your furry friend's diet, whether vegan or otherwise, it is highly recommended to consult with a qualified veterinarian. They possess the proficiency to facilitate a seamless transition for your dog, thereby mitigating any potential digestive distress. Moving forward to a discussion on the enduring well-being of your cherished pet! Although the scientific community is still in the process of elucidating the complete ramifications of vegan nutrition for dogs, several studies suggest that such diets may potentially diminish the likelihood of chronic ailments. Visualize it as an impregnable shield of antioxidants safeguarding your loyal companion!

Let us delve into the scientific aspect (albeit in a more intriguing fashion): fruits, vegetables, and legumes – the crème de la crème in vegan canine sustenance – are replete with antioxidants. These minuscule combatants serve as an invaluable line of defense against free radicals, pernicious entities that possess the capacity to impair your dog's cells and exacerbate the onset of long-term diseases.

Bonus Tip: Berries are like antioxidant ninjas, packed with anthocyanins. Sweet potatoes and carrots? They're beta-carotene bodyguards! With all these plant-powered warriors on your dog's side, their body has a fighting chance against those chronic disease bullies.

Vegan Chow: The Anti-Inflammatory, Weight-Loss Wonder Weapon (For Dogs, Not You)!

We all know that feeling – your dog looks at you with those big, sad eyes, but every time they eat their regular food, it's like Mount Vesuvius erupts in their digestive tract. Yikes! Traditional dog food, with all that meaty goodness, can be a nightmare for sensitive pups. But fear not, pet parents! Vegan dog food might be the superhero cape your canine companion needs! Here's the thing: chronic inflammation can be a real drag for dogs, showing up in everything from itchy allergies to achy joints. Well, some plant-based superstars in vegan food, like turmeric (think a natural pain reliever!), might have some hidden anti-inflammatory superpowers. It is analogous to bestowing upon your canine companion a natural sedative, owing to the miraculous properties bestowed upon us by plants! (However, it behooves us to acknowledge that additional study is requisite, as science is so astutely refined in its pursuits.) It is an undeniable reality that certain canines possess a physique akin to that of tightly wrapped furry casings enveloping a delectable sausage, and this excess weight may precipitate a myriad of health complications. Vegan food, being lower in calorie density than some meat-based options, can be a lifesaver (or should we say, a leash-saver?). Think of it as a diet food for your dog, without the cardboard taste! They'll feel full and satisfied without packing on the pounds, which can help reduce the risk of diabetes, heart disease, and those dreaded joint problems that come with being a chunky monkey.

Now, here's where vegan food gets even cooler: it might be a secret weapon for specific doggy ailments. For pups with kidney troubles, a plant-based diet might be easier on their kidneys compared to a high-protein meat diet. (Please seek guidance from your veterinarian before implementing any alterations in your pet's diet to avoid potential disruption to vital bodily functions!) Furthermore, recollect those uncomfortable flare-ups stemming from allergic reactions to certain food items. The adoption of a vegan diet, free from animal-derived protein allergens, may provide a viable solution in alleviating your dog's discomfort (and afford respite to your furnishings from incessant scratching).

Warning: The immediate adoption of a tofu-based diet for your dog may elicit unforeseen gastrointestinal disturbances.

Therefore, it is imperative to engage in dialogue with your veterinarian before initiating any dietary modifications, be they vegan or otherwise. By doing so, one may effectively navigate a seamless transition to mitigate the risk of adverse digestive reactions. Although ongoing scientific research on vegan dog nutrition remains at a nascent stage, the potential advantages are undeniably commendable! Embracing a plant-based diet for your canine companion could potentially yield a marked improvement in their overall well-being. Just remember to consult your vet and maybe invest in some chew toys (because even with a healthier diet, some dogs just gotta gnaw on something!).

The discourse at hand revolves around the topic of Eco-Pooch Power, specifically delving into how Vegan Chow, a plant-based diet for canines, can elevate both you and your dog to the esteemed status of environmentally conscious individuals. Allow us to broach the subject of your canine companion's posterior region and the unexpected repercussions it has on our planet. It may come as a revelation to you, dear reader, that conventional dog food, brimming with delectable meaty substances, carries with it a substantial ecological footprint. However, fret not, for ethically aware pet guardians! Vegan dog food emerges as a potent solution, offering a pathway towards a more sustainable and prosperous existence for both our furry friends and the Earth at large. It is plausible that adopting a vegan diet for your dog could serve as the pivotal factor in fostering a more harmonious relationship with our environment, potentially yielding a less malodorous outcome for your cherished canine companion. The crux of the matter lies in the formidable domain of agribusiness, where the relentless demand for meat products exerts a colossal strain on our natural resources. One need only consider the alarming rate at which vast expanses of forests are razed to the ground to accommodate the production of beef and poultry, a process that unfolds with such rapidity that it rivals the swiftness of a squirrel darting through the undergrowth. This deforestation thing is a big no-no for wildlife and just makes the whole planet look a little less like a rainforest paradise.

Then there's the water-guzzling. Raising livestock takes a ton of water, way more than growing those yummy peas and lentils that go into vegan dog food. Think of it as giving your pup a built-in water conservation system – they eat, and the planet breathes a sigh of relief! And let's not forget the greenhouse gas party. Livestock farming throws a massive bash, spewing out methane gas like there's no tomorrow. This methane is a real climate change bully, warming things up way faster than we'd like. Vegan food, on the other hand, is a much calmer guest, keeping the greenhouse gas party under control.

So, how does vegan dog food turn your pup into an eco-warrior? Here's the positive side:

Land Saved = Happy Trees: Plant-based protein sources don't need nearly as much space as all those furry friends. This means more trees get to stay put, which makes everyone happy, especially those cuddly koalas.

Water Warriors: Growing plants for dog food uses way less water than raising livestock. It's like giving your dog a built-in drought-fighting superpower!

Climate Change Champs: Vegan food production keeps the greenhouse gas party to a minimum. Your pup can feel good about doing their part to save the planet, one kibble at a time!

But wait, there's more! Vegan dog food goes beyond just being good for the planet. It can also align with your values:

The Vegan Vibe: If you're already rocking a vegan lifestyle, vegan dog food lets your furry friend join the party. It's like a matching eco-friendly outfit for you and your pup!

Compassionate Companionship: Vegan food lets you extend your love for animals to your four-legged friend. It's like saying, "Hey pup, we're a team that cares about all creatures great and small!"

Remember, every step towards sustainability counts. By choosing vegan dog food, you and your pup can become eco-warriors, tree-hugging champions, and all-around good citizens of the planet. Just don't forget the poop bags – eco-friendly ones, of course!

Chapter 4

Crafting Delicious and Nutritious Vegan Meals

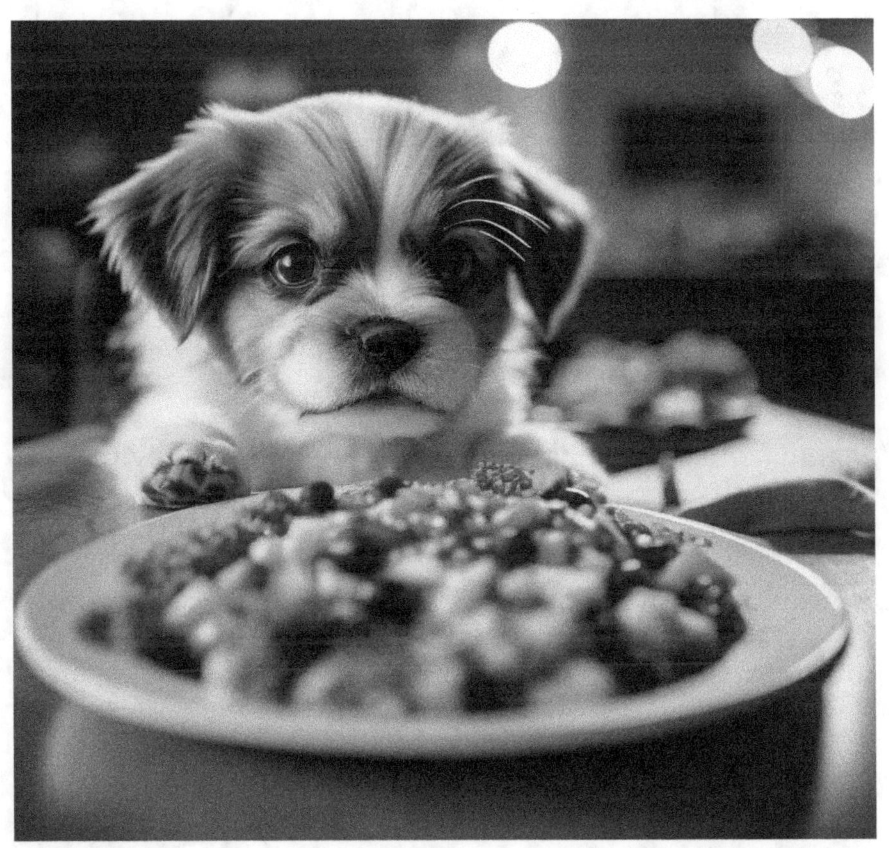

Unleash Your Inner Canine Chef (But Call Your Vet First!)

Let's face it, store-bought kibble can be, well, kibble-ing. Sure, those fancy brands with pictures of Alpenglow mountains and frolicking huskies promise a balanced diet, but where's the *pizzazz*? In this chapter, we'll whip up some drool-worthy (and hopefully vet-approved) vegan meals for your pup, turning dinner time into a five-course tail-wagging affair.

Hold Your Horses (or Leashes): Consult Your Vet First!

Before you swap kibble for kale chips, a chat with your veterinarian is key. They're basically doggy dieticians, ensuring your pup gets all the nutrients to grow from a tiny ankle-biter into a majestic (vegan) mastadon.

Danger Zone: Foods Your Pup Should Avoid

Not everything that's good for you is good for Fido. We're talking grapes that could turn into grape-fruitful trips to the emergency vet, and onions that might leave your pup crying (not tears of joy). Researching vegan dog-friendly ingredients is crucial. Trust me, you don't want to be the one who accidentally turned your poodle into a pickle (unless it's a *very* cute pickle).

Supplements: The Secret Sauce (That Isn't Actually Sauce)

Homemade meals are fantastic, but they often lack the pre-packaged goodness of, well, a package. Work with your vet to find doggy-licious supplements that fill in any nutritional gaps.

Start Slow: From Kibble Kadet to Vegan Viking

Introducing new foods is like playing doggy roulette with digestion. Go slow, and monitor your pup's, ahem, "output" for any signs of distress. Remember, a happy gut equals a happy butt-wiggle.

Okay, Okay, Enough Talk, Let's Get Cooking!

While pre-made vegan dog food might be the ultimate convenience, here are some sample meals to inspire your inner canine chef. Remember, this is just a starting point – always consult your vet for a personalized doggy dining plan!

Sample Meals for Growing Pups (Ages 6 months to 1 year)

Puppies are like furry furnaces, needing tons of protein and calories to fuel their incredible growth spurts.

- **Breakfast of Champions:** Think "smashed chickpea scramble" – cooked lentils or chickpeas with brown rice, veggie confetti (carrots, peas, hold the onions!), a drizzle of flaxseed oil (for that shiny coat!), and a sprinkle of vet-approved puppy vitamins.

- **Dinnertime Delight:** Picture a "quinoa power bowl" with crumbled tofu (think doggy tempeh!), steamed sweet potato for extra sweetness, chopped greens (spinach or kale, because they're like Popeye for pups!), and a sprinkle of that magic vitamin B12 supplement.

Adult Dog (Ages 1-7 years old): The Athlete (Who Secretly Dreams of a Nap)

Your adult dog is basically a canine Olympian (minus the whole opposable thumbs thing). They burn through energy like nobody's business, so we need to keep those engines fueled.

- **Breakfast of Champions (But Make it Oatmeal):** Picture this – a steaming bowl of "oatmeal power porridge" with mashed banana (potassium for all that paw-some jumping!), chia seeds (because chia!), a drizzle of coconut oil (for that beach-bum sheen), and a sprinkle of multivitamin sprinkles (because nobody likes a foggy-brained doggy).

- **Dinnertime Feast:** Imagine a hearty "veggie lentil soup-er bowl" (made with safe veggies, none of that suspicious onion business) with fluffy brown rice and a sprinkle of taurine dust (to keep those peepers sharp).

Senior Dog (7 years and older): The Wise Old Pup (Who May Need Dinner Cut Up)

Senior pups are like the Yoda of the dog world. Full of wisdom, maybe a little stiff in the mornings, and possibly needing their food cut up into bite-sized pieces.

- **Breakfast for the Distinguished Gentleman/Lady:** Think "deluxe kibble soak" – take some store-bought (because convenience is king!) vegan kibble, drench it in pumpkin puree (for extra digestive zen), add a dollop of plain, lactose-free yogurt (because probiotics are all the rage, even for doggos), and sprinkle with a dash of glucosamine magic (check with your vet first, it's like doggy super glue for their joints!).

- **Dinner for the Refined Palate:** Picture a "sophisticated cottage cheese cobbler" – mix unsalted cottage cheese with cooked sweet potato (because sweet potatoes are like doggy antioxidant bombs!), add chopped cooked chicken breast (optional, for an extra protein punch!), and sprinkle with a senior multivitamin medley (again, clear it with your vet).

Treat Time: DIY Doggie Delights (Because Who Doesn't Love a Snack?)

Homemade treats are like doggy ice cream – fun, delicious, but gotta keep it healthy and occasional. Here are some ideas to get your inner canine chef going:

- **Frozen Banana Bonanza:** Mash a ripe banana and freeze it in small cubes for a refreshing summer treat that'll have your pup saying " YUM!"
- **Baked Apple Chips:** Slice apples into thin rounds, bake them on low heat until dehydrated, and voila! A crunchy and healthy snack that'll make your pup feel like a sophisticated chipmunk.

- **Sweet Potato Sizzle Sticks:** Cut sweet potatoes into thin sticks, bake them with a sprinkle of cinnamon, and let them cool for a delicious and nutritious treat that's sweet without the sugar overload.

Remember, these are just a springboard for your creativity. Portion sizes will vary depending on your dog's age, breed, and activity level. But most importantly, always listen to your vet – they're the ultimate authority on all things canine cuisine. With a little planning and some vet wisdom, you can whip up delicious and nutritious meals that'll have your dog wagging their tail and thanking their lucky stars (or should we say lucky kibble?) for such a pawsome pet parent!

Canine Cuisine 101: How to Turn Your Pup into a Foodie (Without Needing a Loan for Truffle Oil)

So, you've graduated from kibble kindergarten and are ready to whip up some gourmet grub for your furry friend. But hold on to your whisks – unlike us fancy humans, dogs don't exactly have Michelin-star taste buds. This chapter will unleash the secret ingredients to creating meals that are both drool-worthy and good for your pup's well-being.

Decoding Doggy Dinners: It's Not All About Fancy Flavors

Let's face it, Fido isn't exactly a connoisseur of caviar. Unlike us, dogs have a more limited taste bud party going on. They can mainly detect sweet, salty, bitter, and sour flavors. Umami (that savory goodness) is there too, but kind of like a shy guest at a doggy dinner party.

The Nose Knows (Especially When It Comes to Dinner):

What dogs *do* have going for them is a nose that could put a bloodhound to shame. Think of it as their built-in food critic. Strong, enticing smells are what get their tails wagging at mealtime. So, fresh ingredients with powerful aromas are your secret weapon.

Flavor Hacks for Happy Eaters:

- **Herbs are Your Pup's New BFFs:** Think of them as doggy breath mints with a bonus! Parsley, rosemary, and basil (in small amounts!) can add a delightful "what-is-this-magical-smell?" factor to your recipes. Just remember to introduce them slowly and see how your pup reacts.

- **Fruity Fun (in Moderation):** While fruits shouldn't be a main course, a little mashed banana, some blueberries, or chopped apples can add a touch of sweetness and an enticing aroma. Just make sure you choose dog-safe options and skip anything with pits or seeds.

- **Vegetable Medley: Let the Colors Shine!:** Think of veggies as edible confetti for your pup's bowl. Roasted sweet potatoes, steamed broccoli florets, or mashed butternut squash can add exciting textures, flavors, and a healthy dose of nutrients. Remember, always cook vegetables thoroughly before feeding them to your dog.

- **Spice Up Their Life (But Not Too Much!):** A pinch of cinnamon or turmeric (always check with your vet first!) can add a subtle warmth or earthiness to your recipes. But remember, strong spices like garlic and onion are a big no-no for dogs – they're like doggy kryptonite!

Balancing Flavor with Fun: Because Who Wants Bland Bean Gruel?

Okay, so you've mastered the doggy dinner party basics, but a truly pawsome meal needs more than just colorful veggies. We need to address the main course – the protein powerhouses that keep your pup feeling like a superhero (without the questionable cape).

- **Legume Lovefest:** Think of lentils and chickpeas as the Dwayne "The Rock" Johnsons of the bean world – the foundation of a strong vegan meal. Mash them up, lightly brown them (think doggy popcorn!), or get creative! Just remember, variety is the spice of life (though avoid actual spice, we'll get to that later).

- **Carb Chaos (But the Good Kind):** Whole grains like brown rice and quinoa are basically doggy jet fuel. They provide complex carbohydrates for sustained energy, meaning your pup can zoom around the house like a furry tornado for longer. Mixing these cooked grains with mashed veggies adds some fun texture – like a built-in doggy sensory playground in their bowl!

- **Healthy Fat Frenzy: A Drizzle of Deliciousness:** Flaxseed oil or coconut oil are like doggy beauty products and energy boosters in a bottle. A drizzle adds healthy fats and makes the whole meal smell amazing (important, because remember, doggy super sniffer!). These fats also contribute to a shiny coat, so your pup will be ready to turn heads (and maybe steal some admiring belly rubs) at the park.

But Wait, There's More!

- **Vet First, Feast Later:** Always get your vet's thumbs up before introducing anything new to your dog's diet, even herbs or spices. They're basically doggy dieticians, making sure your pup gets all the good stuff.

- **Slow and Steady Wins the Race (Especially When It Comes to Tummies):** Introduce new ingredients gradually to avoid any digestive distress. Think of it as a doggy taste test – monitor their reaction and adjust the recipe as needed. Nobody wants a gassy pup (except maybe other dogs, but that's a conversation for another walk).

- **Presentation is Pawsome!:** Even the most delicious meal can be a turn-off if it looks like yesterday's news. Warm the food slightly before serving, and consider using a food puzzle or snuffle mat. Think of it as a doggy treasure hunt for dinner – keeps them mentally stimulated and makes mealtime more fun!

By understanding your dog's preferences and using these tips, you can create flavorful and balanced vegan meals that are both nutritious and enjoyable. Remember, homemade meals are like doggy appetizers – a delicious complement to a well-formulated commercially prepared vegan dog food. With a little creativity and some vet guidance, you can turn mealtime into a culinary adventure for your pup, nourishing their body and tantalizing their taste buds. Now, let's tackle those picky eaters – because let's face it, some pups are just drama queens (or kings) when it comes to food.

Conquering the Picky Eater: Because Even Pups Can Be Drama Queens (or Kings) When It Comes to Dinner

So, you've crafted a culinary masterpiece – a vegan feast fit for a canine king (or queen). But instead of digging in with gusto, your pup gives you the side-eye and performs the world's most dramatic yawn. Ugh, picky eaters! Before you throw in the towel and order takeout (tempting, we know), let's troubleshoot those finicky taste buds.

Is it Medical or Manners?

First things first – a sudden change in appetite could signal a health issue. A trip to the vet is key to rule out any underlying problems before you blame it on their "refined palate."

Treats? More Like Spoiled Rotten Treats!

If your pup is used to a constant flow of gourmet cheese puffs (we're looking at you, Aunt Linda!), they might be less than thrilled with plain old kibble (or even your lovingly crafted vegan masterpiece). Limit those treats, and focus on offering a balanced vegan diet that'll keep their engine running smoothly.

Neophobia? Don't Even Get Us Started...

Some pups are basically canine curmudgeons – suspicious of anything new, especially food. Patience is your best friend here. Introduce new ingredients slowly, like a doggy food taster introducing them to the latest kale chip trend.

Operation: Entice the Picky Eater

- **The Allure of Aroma:** Think doggy aromatherapy! Boost the scent of your homemade meals with ingredients that have a powerful doggy perfume, like roasted sweet potatoes or a drizzle of (vet-approved, of course) olive oil. Basically, make their nose do the happy dance.

- **The Familiar Favorite Trick:** Add a tiny sprinkle of something your pup already knows and loves, like a bit of shredded chicken (if not strictly vegan) or a dollop of plain yogurt (unsweetened, lactose-free, because doggy lactose intolerance is a real thing). Gradually reduce this over time as your pup gets used to the new flavors.

- **Warm it Up, Baby!:** Cold food? No thank you, says your inner canine. Gently warm their vegan meals before serving. Think doggy comfort food – warm and inviting.

- **Playtime with a Purpose:** Food puzzles and snuffle mats are like doggy brain teasers with a delicious reward at the end (their vegan meal!). This can distract them from focusing solely on the "new and scary" flavors and textures.

- **Patience is a Pawsome Virtue:** Don't force your pup to eat. Picky eating can be a phase, just like their teenage obsession with chewing your favorite shoes. Offer the vegan meal, but remove it after a reasonable time. Fresh water is key, and try again at the next mealtime. Consistency is your secret weapon.

Remember, with a little creativity and these tips, you can turn your pup from a picky eater into a full-fledged vegan connoisseur (well, maybe not a connoisseur, but at least an enthusiastic eater!).

Additional Tips: Because Even Pups Get Bored of the Same Old Tofu Scramble

So, you've mastered the art of picky eater persuasion and your pup is finally chowing down on their vegan victuals. But hold your horses (or leashes) – just like us, canines crave a little culinary variety. Here's how to keep things interesting for those furry taste buds:

- **Spice Up Their Life (But Not Literally!):** Rotate different protein sources like lentils, chickpeas, or even the occasional (vet-approved) veggie burger to keep things exciting. Think of it as a doggy world food tour – one day they're feasting on lentil bolognese, the next they're savoring a chickpea curry.

- **Veggie Variety Pack:** Don't let your pup become a broccoli bore. Swap out those steamed florets for some roasted sweet potato cubes or a dollop of mashed butternut squash. A colorful veggie medley is like a doggy disco party in their bowl – exciting, vibrant, and full of good stuff!

- **Setting the Mood (Because Ambiance Matters, Even for Pups):** Think doggy fine dining – a calm and quiet environment for mealtime. No loud noises, no wrestling with the neighbor's poodle over a tennis ball. Just your pup, their food, and the promise of a delicious and nutritious vegan feast.

- **Positive Reinforcement: You Got This!:** When your pup takes a bite (or, ideally, polishes off their entire meal!), shower them with praise and maybe even a (healthy) doggy treat. Positive reinforcement is like doggy psychology 101 – it helps create a happy association with their new vegan grub.

Remember, transitioning your dog to a new diet is a marathon, not a sprint. Be patient, experiment with different flavors and textures, and of course, consult your vet if you have any questions. With a little time and persistence, your pup might just become the envy of the dog park, happily chomping down on their vegan meals while other pups drool over kibble. Now that's a pawsome accomplishment!

Chapter 5

MAKING VEGAN DOG FOOD WORK FOR YOUR LIFESTYLE

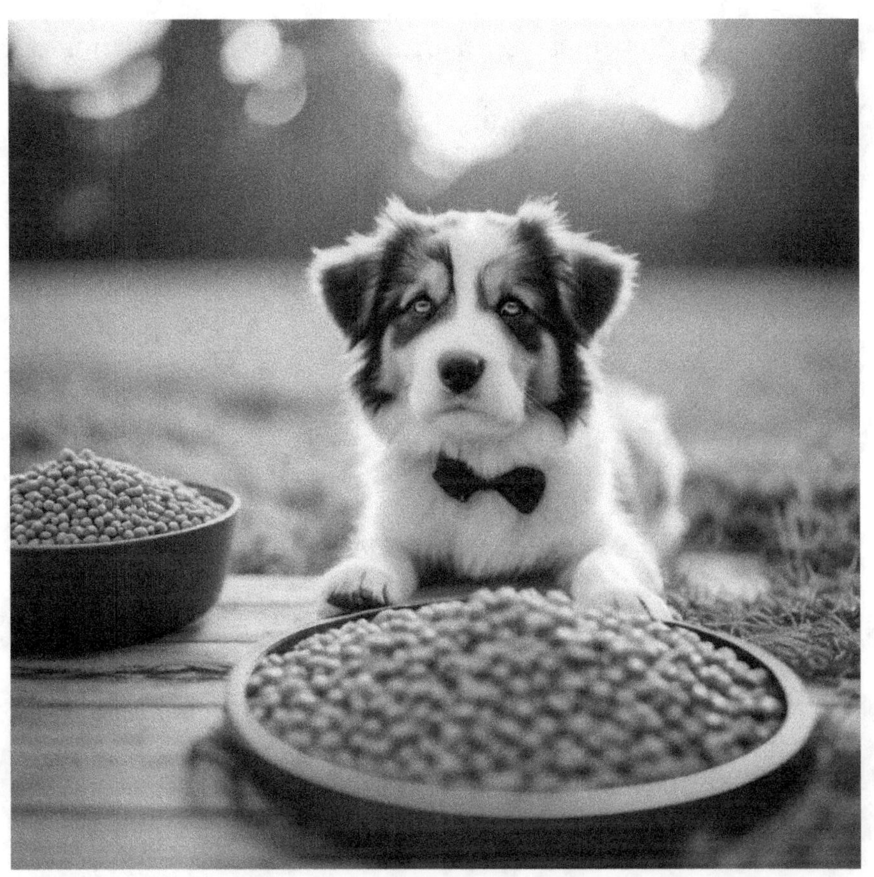

Meal Prep Strategies for Busy Dog Owners

Let's face it, fellow pet parents, between chasing our tails (metaphorically, of course) and dodging drool missiles, whipping up gourmet vegan meals for our furry friends can feel like wrangling a squirrel with a spork. But fear not, because this chapter is here to turn your kitchen into a canine-approved prep station without derailing your busy schedule.

- **Planning Like a Pugilist:**

First things first: we gotta strategize. Think of it as scouting your opponent before a dog park showdown. Dedicate some quality time (translation: don't get attacked by laundry) to plan your pup's meals. Consider their age, activity level, and any dietary quirks they might have (picky eaters, we feel you). The internet is your oyster (or should we say, "lentil"?), so scour the web for drool-worthy recipes or snag a cookbook specifically designed for vegan doggy delights.

Here's the secret weapon: **bulk cooking**. Think of yourself as a canine cafeteria chef. Whip up a vat of lentil stew or a chickpea extravaganza over the weekend. Portion those bad boys out and freeze them for easy access throughout the week. The same goes for brown rice and quinoa – consider them your pup's sidekicks. Wash, chop, and store dog-safe veggies like carrots, broccoli, or sweet potatoes in advance. Trust us, future you will thank yourself when you're dodging dodgeball-sized kibble at 7 am.

Meal Prep Magic: From Fridge to Fido in Minutes

- **Breakfast of Champions (Canine Edition):** The night before, soak a portion of pre-cooked oatmeal in warm water, like prepping for a marathon snuggle session. In the morning, throw in some mashed banana (bonus points for using one that looks like a dog bone!), a drizzle of flaxseed oil (because why not be fancy?), and a sprinkle of vet-approved supplements. Your pup will be begging for this breakfast of champions before you can say "walkies."

- **Leftovers for the Win:** Cooking a vegan stir-fry for yourself? Don't forget your furry sous chef! Set aside a portion without the extra salt and spices for your dog. Combine it with some pre-cooked brown rice or quinoa for a lunch that's both nutritious and faster than a squirrel up a tree.

- **Dinnertime Delight:** Thaw a portion of those pre-cooked lentils or chickpeas, mash them with a fork (because who has time for fancy food processors?), and combine them with some prepped veggies and a drizzle of coconut oil for a satisfying and flavorful dinner. Your pup will be so busy scarfing this down, they won't even notice you haven't gotten around to washing those dishes yet.

Beyond Batch Cooking: Hacks for the Time-Strapped Vegan Pet Parent

So, you've mastered the art of canine cafeteria cooking, but let's be honest, who has all the time in the world? Here's how to keep your pup on the plant-based path without becoming a short-order cook for a very demanding (and furry) customer.

Slow Cooker Shenanigans: Ditch the fancy gadgets and embrace the magic of the slow cooker. Toss in a bunch of veggies, your pup's favorite legume du jour (lentils? chickpeas? Don't worry, they won't judge your culinary creativity), and maybe even a stray sock (hey, it happens!). Let it simmer all day while you're busy conquering the world (or at least conquering that mountain of laundry). Dinner will be ready when you are, and your house will smell like a gourmet vegan doggy spa (minus the actual spa treatments, because let's face it, Fido might shed everywhere).

Subscription Box Bonanza: Feeling fancy? Explore subscription services that deliver pre-portioned, frozen vegan dog food meals straight to your door. Think of it like takeout for your pup, but way healthier (and probably less likely to come with a side of fortune cookie wisdom your dog can't decipher). Plus, you get to feel smug about being a super-efficient pet parent, even if the real hero is the delivery person.

Teamwork Makes the Dream Work (and the Kibble Disappear): Living with a roommate or significant other who (hopefully) doesn't mind sharing their kitchen with a canine connoisseur of plant-based cuisine? Divide and conquer! One person can be the "bean brigade" general, whipping up lentil stews fit for a doggy king, while the other becomes the "chop-chop champion," transforming vegetables into bite-sized doggy delights. Working together cuts down on prep time and might even lead to some hilarious kitchen mishaps that will make for epic pet-parent stories later.

Important Side Quests: Safety First (and Always!)

Remember, even though your pup might have the begging skills of a master thespian, food safety is paramount. Wash your hands and surfaces like a pro to prevent any bacterial villains from crashing your dog's next dinner party.

Portion Patrol: Just because your homemade meals are plant-based doesn't mean they're a free pass for your pup to become a blimp. Talk to your vet to figure out the perfect amount of food for your furry friend, because even the healthiest vegan treats can lead to a situation where your dog looks more like a fluffy potato than a sleek canine athlete.

Fresh is the best: While freezing ingredients is a lifesaver, whenever possible, offer your dog a variety of fresh fruits and veggies alongside their prepped meals. Think of it as a doggy salad bar – it adds some excitement to their diet and gives them a chance to practice their foraging skills (minus the actual digging in the backyard, hopefully).

Traveling with your Vegan Pup! Buckle up, because we're about to embark on an adventure to ensure your furry friend has a smooth journey and doesn't miss out on their plant-powered meals.

Planning and Preparation:

So, you and your furry friend are ready to hit the road, but your pup's plant-based diet has you worried about becoming a kibble-smuggling bandit? Fear not, intrepid pet parent! Here's how to ensure your vegan pup has a adventure without resorting to questionable gas station hot dog purchases (for them, at least).

Finding Fido-Friendly Fun: Just because your dog prefers tempeh over tripe doesn't mean your vacation options are kibble-sized. Research pet-friendly destinations with restaurants or stores that offer vegan options. Think "charming cafes with pupcakes" or "vegan food truck rallies" – your pup will thank you (with lots of tail wags, hopefully, less drool). Many travel websites and apps let you filter accommodations and restaurants based on pet-friendliness and vegan options, so you can become a travel ninja who finds the perfect spot for both you and your furry foodie. Don't tempt fate (or your dog's digestive system) by relying solely on finding vegan dog food at your destination. Pack enough of their regular food to last the entire trip, with a little extra buffer in case of unexpected travel delays. Think of it like packing an insurance policy against a very hangry canine meltdown. Pre-portioning food into travel containers can be a lifesaver, especially if you're more of a "throw everything in a duffel bag and hope for the best" kind of packer (no judgment here).

- **Paperwork Pointers (Because Border Collies Don't Carry Passports)**

If you're jet-setting internationally, some countries might require your pup to have more documents than a secret agent. We're talking health certificates, proof of vaccinations, the whole shebang. Check the entry requirements for your destination well in advance and make sure your dog's paperwork is up-to-date. Nobody wants a "hangry AND grounded" situation at the airport.

- **Hitting the Road: Essentials for the Vegan Pup on the Go**

Bowls of Glory (That Collapse!): Pack collapsible food and water bowls for easy use during pit stops, hikes, or epic sightseeing adventures. Look for bowls made from food-safe, BPA-free materials – because who wants a side of harmful chemicals with their kibble-less kibble? Bring along some familiar and travel-friendly vegan dog treats to reward good behavior and keep your dog occupied during the journey. Think dehydrated fruits like banana chips or apple slices – healthy, portable, and won't make you look like you raided the Smithsonian gift shop for your dog's snacks. If you're planning on dining out with your dog, call restaurants in advance to inquire about their vegan options and if they allow furry patrons on their patios. Imagine the Instagram-worthy photo opportunities: you, sipping a latte, your dog enjoying a tofu scramble – pure #travelgoals.

Home Away from Home (But With More Sniffing Opportunities): Choose pet-friendly hotels or vacation rentals that allow dogs. Some accommodations might even offer amenities like dog walking services or on-site pet relief areas – a dream come true for busy pet parents and pups who need a potty break. Don't forget to pack a familiar blanket, bed, or toy for your dog to help them feel comfortable and secure in a new environment. After all, a happy pup is a travel-ready pup!

- **Keeping Your Pup on a Predictable Poop Schedule (Because Nobody Wants Surprises):** Sticking to your dog's regular feeding schedule and exercise routine during travel is like packing a magic stress shield. Think of it as a preventative measure against digestive meltdowns that would make even the most seasoned traveler green in the gills (and hopefully not your dog).

If you're crossing international borders, be prepared for your dog's food to undergo a full-on customs inspection. Declare the food and have documentation from your vet stating it's a gourmet vegan feast for your furry friend, not a secret stash of questionable snacks. A little paperwork can save you a whole lot of hangry howls at the airport. Being a responsible pet owner is travel rule number one. Always clean up after your dog and dispose of waste properly, because nobody wants to step in a surprise (except maybe a particularly enthusiastic dung beetle). Respect the environment and local regulations, and your pup will be hailed as a travel ambassador (and not a walking biohazard). Traveling with your vegan dog is an adventure, but ensuring they have access to delicious (and tummy-friendly) food requires some serious resourcefulness. Here's how to navigate the world of vegan dog food options without your pup getting hangry: Utilize resources like online pet food retailers or apps that allow you to search for stores offering vegan dog food brands. National pet store chains like Petco or PetSmart might carry vegan options in some locations (it's like playing a game of kibble roulette!). If you're jet-setting internationally, research vegan pet stores or online retailers in your destination city. Don't rely solely on online listings. Call pet stores at your destination or along your travel route to confirm they stock the vegan dog food brands your pup knows and loves. This can save you the time and frustration of showing up to a store with a hopeful face and a hungry dog, only to discover they're fresh out of lentil loaf. Explore subscription services that deliver pre-portioned, shelf-stable vegan dog food to your travel destination. This can be a lifesaver for extended trips, especially if your suitcase is already overflowing with enough dog toys to open a boutique. Think of it as a gourmet doggy room service, minus the tiny white gloves and the hefty bill (hopefully).

Travel Hacks for the Fearless Vegan Pup Parent (Because Kibble Emergencies Are No Fun):

Online Ordering: A Race Against the Hangry Howls: Many online pet food retailers offer lightning-fast shipping options. If you have internet access that isn't slower than a sloth on a sugar crash, and a schedule as flexible as a rubber band, consider ordering vegan dog food directly to your posh hotel (or slightly less posh campground) **before** your current food supply performs a disappearing act. Remember, a hungry pup is a symphony of sad whines and desperate stares – avoid the drama at all costs.

Farmers Markets: Fresh Finds for the Fido Forager: While fresh produce isn't a complete doggy dinner, farmers markets can be a treasure trove of travel-friendly additions to your pup's meals. Think of it as a doggy salad bar on the go! Just remember, not all human food is canine cuisine. Stick to dog-safe fruits and veggies (like blueberries or baby carrots), and always check with your vet about portion sizes – you don't want your pup to turn into a furry bowling ball.

Dehydrated Dog Chow: Lightweight and Ready to Rumble: Dehydrated vegan dog food is the Mary Poppins' purse of kibble – lightweight, compact, and ready for any adventure. Just add water (from your trusty travel water bottle) and voila! Instant doggy dinner. Look for brands with packaging that seals tighter than a clam at high tide to keep things fresh throughout your travels.

Backup Plans and Canine Cuisine SOS:

Carry a Vet's Seal of Approval: Having a veterinarian's recommendation for a top-notch, commercially available vegan dog food brand can be your saving grace if vegan options are rarer than an honest politician. This little cheat sheet can help you chat with pet store staff or vets at your destination who might look at you like you just asked for kangaroo milk (because, let's face it, some people just haven't gotten the vegan pet food memo yet).

Be Open to Exploring Alternative Routes: If finding vegan dog food feels like searching for a unicorn, discuss alternative options with your vet beforehand. They might suggest a temporary switch to a commercially available vegetarian dog food, or maybe a combo of vegetarian food with some strategically chosen vegan supplements to keep your pup getting all the good stuff.

Remember: Your Pup's Health is Pawsomely Important: While finding vegan dog food options on the go can be a challenge, your dog's health is what truly matters. If necessary, be prepared to adjust your plans and consider vet-approved alternatives to ensure your furry friend gets the nutrients they need.

Communication is Key (Because Even Pups Don't Speak Every Language): Clear communication with pet store staff, vets at your destination, and even your accommodation providers can be your secret weapon. The more people you talk to, the more likely you are to find solutions and ensure your dog has access to food that keeps them happy and healthy throughout your travels.

By combining planning, resourcefulness, and open communication, you can navigate the world of vegan dog food options on the go and ensure your furry friend has an epic travel adventure by your side!

Chapter 6

Breakfast Powerhouse Meals to Fuel your Dog's Day

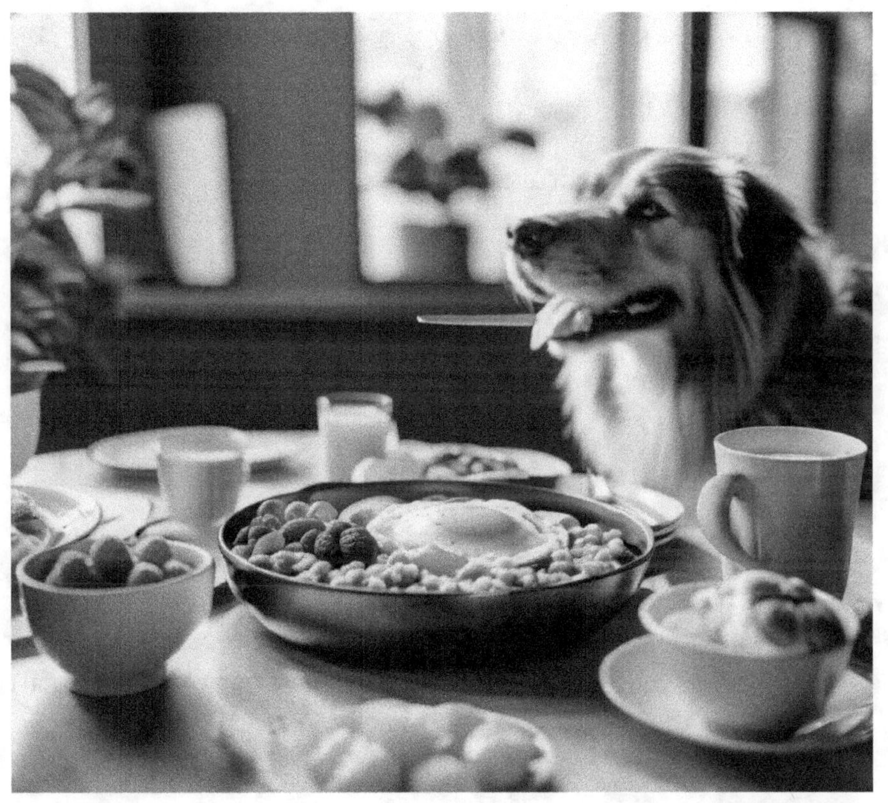

Fueling Fido's Fantastic Feats: A Breakfast Fit for a Canine Conqueror

Forget boring kibble! It's time to whip up a breakfast that'll have your dog ditching their drool-worthy dreams for a drool-worthy reality. This ain't your average bowl of mush – this is the Energetic Quinoa and Veggie Scramble, a culinary masterpiece designed to turn your pup from a sleepy sausage into a furry force of nature!

Ingredients:

- 1 cup cooked quinoa (rinsed beforehand, unless your dog enjoys a gritty adventure)
- ½ cup chopped cooked veggies (broccoli florets the size of tiny trees, carrot coins smaller than their gold-loving namesake, green beans – choose whatever your dog can demolish without resembling a chipmunk)

- ½ cup mashed chickpeas or lentils (because legume love is a real thing, and protein is the key to unlocking epic zoomies)

- 1 tablespoon nutritional yeast (optional, but think of it as doggy B vitamin sprinkles!)

- 1 tablespoon finely chopped fresh parsley (or other herbs your dog won't try to bury in the backyard – basil or rosemary, for the adventurous eater)

- ¼ cup warm water (adjust as needed, depending on your dog's preferred level of sauciness)

- Coconut oil spray (because even breakfast battles require a little non-stick magic)

Instructions:

1. **The Quinoa Quest:** In a saucepan, rinse the quinoa like you're searching for buried treasure (except it's tiny, white, and not treasure). Follow the package

instructions to cook this magic grain, aiming for a texture that's not too crunchy, not too mushy – just right for a happy pup. Let it cool slightly because nobody likes a face-planting breakfast.

2. **Veggie Victory:** Wash those veggies, then unleash your inner Michelangelo and sculpt them into bite-sized masterpieces. Steam or boil them until they're tender enough for even the most challenged chewer. Leftovers from your meals are welcome – who needs fancy dog food stores when you've got a gourmet chef at home (that's you, by the way)?

3. **Chickpea Coronation (or Lentil Lordship):** Grab a separate bowl and transform those chickpeas or lentils into a chunky spread using a fork. Think of it as crafting tiny, edible crowns for your canine king (or queen).

4. **The Breakfast Bonanza:** In a large bowl, gather your cooked quinoa, mashed legumes, veggie creations, optional B vitamin sprinkles, and finely chopped herbs. Mix it all together gently – you don't want to turn this into a dog-gone salsa!

5. **The Sizzling Showdown:** Preheat a non-stick pan on medium heat. Apply a light coat of coconut oil spray to prevent any food from adhering to the surface (with the exception of your admiration for this exceptional breakfast). Now comes the fun part: pour in the quinoa and veggie mixture, spreading it out like a furry pizza.

6. **Patty Power:** Grab your spatula and gently press down on the mixture, forming a magnificent (and slightly loose) patty. Cook it for 2-3 minutes per side, until it's a beautiful golden brown and heated all the way through. If things get a little dry, don't despair! Just add a splash

of warm water while cooking to create a more manageable consistency.

7. **Breakfast Bliss:** Let the scramble cool slightly before presenting it to your furry friend. Break it up into smaller pieces for easier consumption, especially for those pint-sized pup lovers.

Now, watch in amazement as your dog devours this breakfast of champions and prepares to conquer the day with the boundless energy of a furry superhero!

Tips:

- **Don't Be a Kibble Criminal: Portion Patrol for Pups**

Alright, let's talk about portion sizes. We all know that look – those big, pleading eyes that could melt glaciers. But resist the urge to turn your dog into a furry blimp! How much breakfast your pup needs depends on their size, age, and activity level. Are they a lumbering Saint Bernard or a hyperactive Chihuahua? Think of it like a car – a Ferrari needs way more gas than a golf cart. Confused? Consult your vet – they're the experts in preventing doggy doughnuts (that's what we're calling love handles now).

- **Mixing it Up: The Veggie Variety Show**

This recipe is your dog's veggie buffet! Feel free to swap in different cooked veggies like sweet potato (because who doesn't love a little sweetness?), peas (just don't let them turn into tiny green projectiles!), or bell peppers (because every breakfast needs a little color, right?). Just remember, stick to dog-safe options – we don't want any doggy tummy troubles.

- **Leftovers? More Like Leftovers for Champions!**

Don't let this breakfast masterpiece go to waste! This recipe easily doubles or triples for meal prep – perfect for those mornings when you're running late because your dog decided to "borrow" your sock collection again. Leftover scramble can be stored in an airtight container in the fridge for up to 3 days. Just reheat it gently before serving – nobody wants a fridge-cold breakfast unless they're a polar bear (and even then, they might prefer fish).

- **Fresh is the Best: Fruits and Veggies are Nature's Candy (But Way Healthier)**

While this recipe uses cooked ingredients, whenever possible, try to offer your dog fresh fruits and veggies alongside their meals. It's like a doggy vitamin and hydration party in their bowl!

Instructions:

The Berry Blast Smoothie Bowl: Unleash Your Pup's Inner Instagram Foodie

Forget boring kibble! It's time to turn your dog into a social media sensation with the Berry Blast Smoothie Bowl, a breakfast so photogenic, you might need to set up a doggy influencer account.

Step 1: Blend Like a Boss

First, we gotta create the smoothie base. Toss those frozen mixed berries (think blueberries, strawberries, raspberries – a berry explosion!), plant-based milk (almond, oat, coconut – whatever your pup fancies!), and a banana (frozen or fresh, it's all good) into your blender. Blend that bad boy until it's smooth and creamy – like a rockstar milkshake for your furry friend. If things get a little thick, just add a splash of more plant-based milk – you don't want your pup to need a straw!

Step 2: Chia Seed Sprinkle Party

While your blender does its thing, grab some chia seeds and have a sprinkle party on a small plate. Think of them as tiny edible confetti for your masterpiece. If you're feeling fancy and using yogurt, spoon it into a separate bowl – it's like a blank canvas for your artistic pup-gurt masterpiece (though knowing dogs, it might end up more on their fur than in the bowl).

Step 3: Bowl-iful Presentation

Now for the fun part – assembling this beauty! Pour that blended smoothie base into a wide, shallow bowl. Imagine it as a tiny doggy canvas. Feeling decorative? Dip the rim of the bowl into the chia seeds, gently pressing them on to create a fancy border. Or, for the less mess-inclined pup parent, you can just sprinkle those little chia seed sprinkles right on top of the smoothie.

Step 4: Top it Off Like a Champion!

This is where your pup's inner food critic gets to shine! Get creative with the toppings – fresh berries (because, well, berries!), sliced banana (potassium power!), chopped apple (minus the seeds and core, of course!), a sprinkle of shredded coconut (for a tropical twist!), or a teeny tiny dollop of nut butter (xylitol-free peanut or almond, but use it sparingly – it's a treat, not the main course!).

Bonus Tips for the Pawsome Chef:

- **Frozen is the Key:** Frozen fruit makes the smoothie thicker and creamier, perfect for a bowl. Fresh fruit is fine too, but you might need some ice cubes to get that spoon-lickin' good consistency.

- **Ripeness Matters (Kind Of):** Fresh banana? Ripe is best for extra sweetness. Frozen banana? Doesn't matter – frozen bananas are like nature's freezy pops for pups!

- **Portion Patrol for Treats:** Those yummy toppings like nut butter? Treats, not staples. Consult your vet on how much is just right for your pup.

- **Hydration Station:** Don't forget the fresh water on the side! Every meal, even smoothie bowls, needs a good H2O companion.

Important Note: This recipe is like a doggy health spa menu, not a doggy grocery list. Yogurt and nut butter are toppings, not main ingredients. Always check with your vet before introducing new foods to your dog's diet. Now go forth and conquer the world (or at least the living room rug) with your pup's brand-new Instagram-famous smoothie bowl! Just remember, pictures first, then playtime!

Calling All Canine Connoisseurs: Pumpkin Power Pancakes with a PB Drizzle fit for Royalty!

Forget boring kibble, these ain't your average flapjacks! We're talking gourmet breakfasts fit for a furry king (or queen). These Pumpkin Power Pancakes are bursting with pumpkin goodness and a touch of peanut butter that'll have your dog begging for more (well, maybe barking excitedly – same difference).

Ingredients:

- 1 cup cooked and mashed pumpkin (think pumpkin puree, not leftover pie filling – we don't want any sugar crashes here!)

- 1 ripe banana, mashed (because potassium is a pup's best friend)

- 1 ½ cups rolled oats, blitzed into a flour-like consistency (basically oat flour for our canine companions)

- 1 tablespoon of ground flaxseed (mixed with 3 tablespoons of warm water to create a magical gloop)

- 1 teaspoon cinnamon (optional, but adds a touch of autumn spice)

- ¼ cup plain, unsweetened yogurt (optional, for an extra protein punch and moisture boost)

- Coconut oil spray (because even pancakes deserve a little non-stick magic)

For the Optional Peanut Butter Drizzle (because everything is better with peanut butter, almost):

- 2 tablespoons of xylitol-free peanut butter (creamy or chunky, your pup decides!)

1. 1-2 tablespoons of warm water are prescribed to accomplish the ideal sprinkling consistency. Instructions: - Start by mixing the oat flour and cinnamon in a huge bowl. - In a different bowl, join the squashed banana, pumpkin puree, and yogurt whenever wanted, until a smooth consistency is accomplished. -

Tenderly overlap the wet fixings into the dry blend to make a thick hitter, like flapjack player however somewhat thicker. Add water on a case by case basis to arrive at the ideal consistency. - Heat a non-stick container over medium intensity, softly lubed with coconut oil. Pour ¼ cup of player onto the skillet, passing on space between every hotcake to take into account spreading. - Cook for 2-3 minutes on each side, or until flapjacks are a brilliant earthy colored tone and completely cooked.. Utilize your spatula to delicately flip them - think about it like a hotcake artful dance!

2. **The Optional PB Drizzle Drama:** If you're feeling extra fancy (and your pup deserves it!), whip up the peanut butter drizzle. In a small bowl, whisk together the peanut butter and warm water until it's smooth and drizzly. You might need to adjust the water depending on how chunky your peanut butter is.

Serving Suggestions:

- Serve these pumpkin masterpieces warm or at room temperature.

- Drizzle that optional peanut butter sauce on top, like a beautiful, nutty crown.

- Or, for the less messy pups, serve a small dollop of peanut butter on the side as a separate treat.

Top Tips:

- **Watch the Clock:** Cooking time can vary depending on how thick your pancakes are. So keep an eye on them to avoid any burning mishaps.

- **Portion Patrol:** How many pancakes your pup gets depends on their size and activity level. Consult your vet for the perfect serving size, because even delicious things come in moderation.

- **Fresh is Best:** While this recipe uses mashed banana, consider offering your dog a small slice of fresh banana on the side for some extra hydration and potassium (because a healthy pup is a happy pup!).

These Pumpkin Power Pancakes with Peanut Butter Drizzle are a delightful combo of flavors and textures that will have your dog wagging their tail with glee. It's a fun twist on breakfast that's perfect for a special occasion or just because your pup deserves a gourmet meal. Remember, always check with your veterinarian before introducing any new foods to your dog's diet. Now go forth and create a breakfast masterpiece your pup will never forget (or at least until dinner)!

Chapter 7

WHOLESOME LUNCH AND DINNER RECIPES FOR OPTIMAL HEALTH

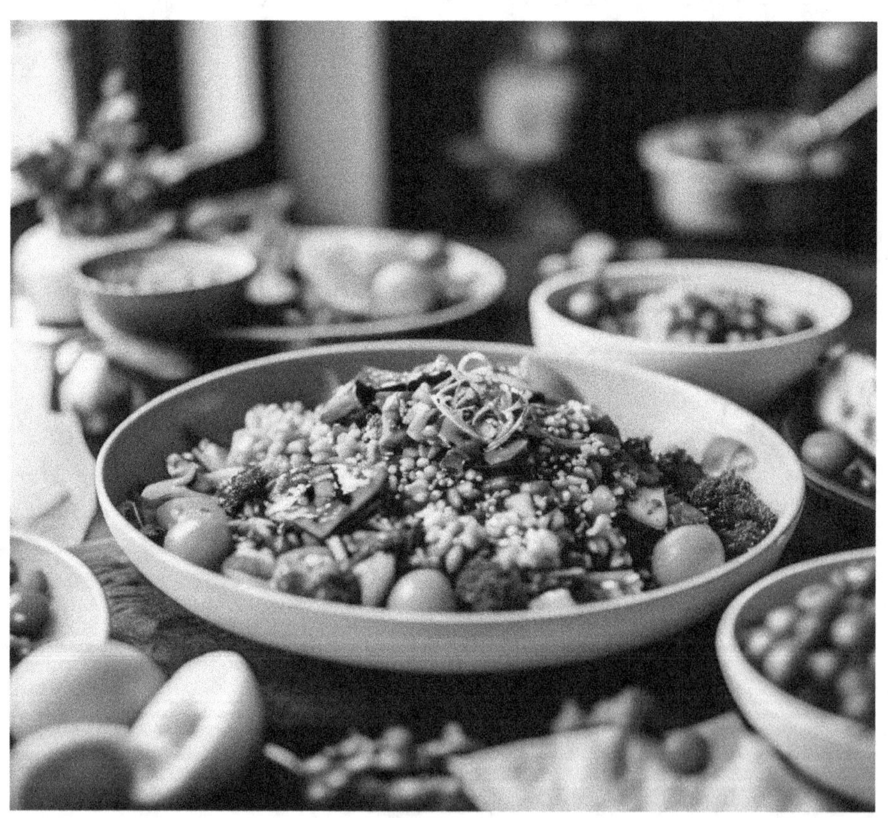

Calling All Canine Connoisseurs: A Gourmet Grub Guide for the Discerning Doggo

This chapter cracks open the doggy dining dilemma, presenting a two-course extravaganza designed to tantalize your tail-wagger's taste buds and keep them zooming like a furry rocket on a plant-powered propellant. We kick things off with a classic comfort dish reimagined for our four-legged foodies: The Lentil Shepherd's Pie with a Brown Rice Crust – because even pups deserve a touch of culinary flair (and hey, maybe it'll trick you into eating your vegetables too!).

Ingredients:

For the Lentil Landfill (Yes, That's What We're Calling It):

- 1 cup brown lentils, rinsed (think of them as tiny, earthy gumballs)

- 2 cups vegetable broth (low-sodium, because woof, too much salt!)

- 1 tablespoon olive oil (for a little lubrication, those lentils can be stubborn)

- 1 medium onion, chopped (because every good doggy dish needs a little sniff-tastic onion action)

- 2 carrots, slashed (on the grounds that beta-carotene for good young men and young ladies!) 1 chopped celery stalk (goodness gracious for those choppers) 1 cup chopped frozen peas (similar to tiny green treasure balls or dog food kibble, depending on how your dog sees it)

- 1 clove garlic, minced (optional, check with your vet first, some pups have sensitive tummies to this fragrant flower)

- ½ teaspoon dried thyme (because fancy herbs elevate even the most basic lentil situation)

- ¼ teaspoon dried rosemary (because every shepherd's pie needs a touch of Earthy Majesty)

- Salt and pepper to taste (consult your veterinarian first, some pups like bland things, weirdos)

For the Brown Rice Roof (Because Every Pie Needs a Top):

- 1 cup cooked brown rice (hearty and healthy, just like your pup!)

- ½ cup mashed sweet potato (because sweetness is happiness for furry friends)

- ¼ cup rolled oats (because texture is everything, even in dog food!)

- 1 tablespoon ground flaxseed (mixed with 3 tablespoons of warm water to create a gel – it's like doggy glue to hold that roof on tight!)

Instructions:

Lentil Landfill Extravaganza:

Put the rinsed lentils and vegetable broth in a pot for the Great Lentil Lagoon. Heat it to the point of boiling like a pup jacuzzi, then, at that point, stew with the top on for 20-25 minutes. You want the lentils to be so soft that even a novice chewer can mash them. Since nobody wants a soupy landfill, drain any liquid that remains. Veggie Bonanza: In a pan, heat some olive oil while your lentils simmer. Throw in that slashed onion, carrot, and celery - let them sauté until they're delicate enough for a pup drum solo. Brighten up Your Little guy's Life: Add that garlic (assuming your vet endorses), thyme, and rosemary. Allow it to sizzle briefly, delivering every one of those awesome pup supported fragrances. The Terrific Lentil and Veggie Get-together: Dump those cooked lentils and frozen peas into the dish with the veggie team. Combine everything and heat through for a few minutes. Salt and pepper to taste (but consult your veterinarian first, as some pups have bland palates).

Brown Rice Roof: The Not-So-Thatched Conclusion

Sweet Potato Squashtacular: Grab that cooked sweet potato and mash it like you're making doggy disco sweet potato fries! Make sure it's smooth, like a dance floor after a good paw-ty.

The Crumbly Crew: Dump your cooked brown rice, rolled oats, and that flaxseed goop (we told you it was like doggy glue!) into the mashed sweet potato. Mash it all together until it forms a thick, slightly sticky mess – think doggy Play-Doh (but way tastier).

Assemble and Bake: The Grand Canine Cuisine Finale

Preheat the Oven to Broil Mode (Just Kidding... Mostly): Set your oven to 375°F (pretend it's a fancy doggy spa day with a heated towel).

Fill 'Er Up: Scoop that lentil filling into a baking dish – think doggy swimming pool, but with food instead of water (because, ew).

The Great Brown Rice Roof Application: Spread that brown rice mush over the top of the filling like a doggy snow cone – but way more filling and way less brain freeze. Press it down gently to make sure it sticks.

Bake It Like You Bark It: Pop that shepherd's pie in the oven for 20-25 minutes. You want that roof to be slightly golden brown, like a perfectly toasted doggy biscuit.

Serving Suggestions:

- Let that shepherd's pie cool down a bit – you don't want your pup to burn their tongue (unless they, you know, stole your slippers again).

- Cut it up into doggy-sized portions – because even the fanciest pups deserve a meal they can manage.

- Double or triple this recipe if you're feeling generous (or have a particularly hungry pup). Leftovers can live in an airtight container in the fridge for up to 3 days. Reheat them gently before serving, because nobody likes cold doggy disco fries.

Tips From the Top Dog Chef:

- **Veggie Variety Hour:** Feel free to throw in different chopped veggies to the lentil filling! Bell peppers, zucchini, green beans – anything your pup can handle and your vet approves of.

- **Fresh is Fetch:** This recipe uses cooked stuff, but consider giving your pup a side salad of fresh greens or chopped veggies for some extra hydration and vitamins. They might not love it, but a good doggy parent provides a balanced meal (and maybe a cuddle afterwards to make up for it).

- **Ask Your Vet About Garlic:** If you gotta add garlic, check with your vet first. Some pups have sensitive tummies, and garlic can be a bit much for them.

This Lentil Shepherd's Pie with Brown Rice Roof is basically a doggy health and happiness explosion in a baking dish. Packed with protein, fiber, and all that good stuff, it's the perfect vegan lunch or dinner for your furry best friend. Now go forth and conquer the kitchen, top chef!

Calling All Canine Chili Fiends: A Stewtastic Spectacular for Dinnertime!

Does your pup get the zoomies when the weather turns into cuddle puddle season? This hearty Chickpea and Sweet Potato Stew will have them howling with glee – and it's not just for chilly days! This pawsome recipe is so versatile, you can serve it up year-round and keep your canine companion coming back for more.

Ingredients:

- 1 tablespoon olive oil (because even healthy food needs a little lubrication)

- 1 medium onion, chopped (sniff-tastic and essential for any self-respecting stew)

- 2 cloves garlic, minced (warning: may lead to extra doggy kisses)

- 1 teaspoon ground cumin (because exotic spices are the new kibble on the block)

- ½ teaspoon ground coriander (another fancy way to say "doggy spice")

- 1/4 teaspoon turmeric (optional, for an extra health kick – but consult your vet first, some pups have sensitive insides)

- Pinch of red pepper flakes (optional, adjust based on your dog's spice tolerance – some pups like things fiery, others prefer bland like a beige carpet)

- 2 cups vegetable broth (low-sodium, because woof, salt!)

- 1 cup chopped sweet potato (like tiny orange treasure troves)

- 1 (15-ounce) can chickpeas, drained and rinsed (because chickpeas are like tiny legume beanie babies... and yes, we know that's weird)

- 2 cups chopped kale, ribs removed and leaves roughly chopped (because leafy greens are good for a pup's insides, even if they look like someone sneezed in the pot)

- ½ cup cooked brown rice or quinoa (optional, for those pups who like a little extra something-something in their stew)

- Fresh parsley or cilantro, chopped (optional, for garnish – mostly to make it look purty for the doggy Instagram)

Instructions:

Sauté the Sniff-Inducing Scents: In a large pot, heat the olive oil and toss the chopped onion in. Sauté it until it's delicate and clear, similar to a pup phantom (however way less startling). Then add the garlic, cumin, coriander, turmeric (in the event that you're utilizing it), and red pepper chips (assuming your little guy likes things zesty). It should be allowed to sizzle for a minute to release all of the delicious aromas that will make your dog drool like a dripping faucet. Broth & Veggie Bonanza: Add the vegetable broth and simmer it, like a gentle dog jacuzzi. The chopped sweet potato and those chickpea beanie babies should then be added. Allow it to simmer for 15 to 20 minutes, or until the sweet potato is soft enough for even the most inexperienced chewer to mash it.

The Kale Prank: Cook the chopped kale for an additional five minutes, or until it wilts like a tired dog after a long walk.

Brown Rice or Quinoa Extravaganza (Optional): If you're feeling fancy, add some cooked brown rice or quinoa for the last minute of cooking.

Serving and Garnish (Optional): Let the stew cool down a bit so your pup doesn't burn their tongue (unless they, you know, ate your favorite shoes again). Dish it out into bowls and if you're feeling extra fancy, sprinkle on some chopped parsley or cilantro. But really, your pup will probably just gobble it up regardless – because stew this good needs no fancy frills!

Top Dog Chef Tips: Spoiler Alert - They Involve Leftovers!

Meal Prep Mumbo Jumbo: This stew is a champion of leftovers! Cook a ton and shove the extras in an airtight container in the fridge for up to 3 days. Reheat it gently before serving, because nobody likes fridge-temperature stew, not even a dog who stole your underwear this morning (no judgment).

Frozen Kale Frenzy: Feeling lazy? Frozen chopped kale is your friend! Just toss it in frozen with the broth and veggies – no shame in the convenience game!

Spice Up Your Pup's Life (But Not Too Much): The red pepper flakes are optional, and frankly, a gamble. Start with a pinch, see how your pup reacts, because some pups like their food like they like their toys – completely squeakless.

Chickpea Chickpeas? No Way! Don't have chickpeas, or worse, your pup has a chickpea allergy? No sweat! Just sub in cooked lentils or kidney beans in equal amounts. But be sure to consult your vet before introducing any new legume to your pup's diet – gotta keep those doggy tummies happy!

Fresh is Fetch (But Cooked Works Too): This recipe is all about the cooked stuff, but consider giving your pup a side of steamed green beans or chopped broccoli for some extra vitamins and hydration. They might not love it, but hey, a good doggy parent provides a balanced meal (and maybe a belly rub afterwards to make up for it).

The Stew-pendous Finale: This Chickpea and Sweet Potato Stew is basically a doggy health and happiness explosion in a pot. It's packed with protein, fiber, and all that good stuff, and it's both versatile and delicious. Serve it on its own, over rice, or frankly, on your head if your pup gets too demanding. Just kidding... mostly.

The Tofu Scramble: Not Your Average Breakfast for Your Canine Connoisseur

Ever wished your dog could join you for brunch? Well, with this Tofu Scramble recipe, they practically can! This dish is a vegan superstar in the human world, and guess what? Pups can get in on the action too.

Base Recipe: The Classic Canine Scramble That Puts Kibble to Shame

Ingredients:

- 1 Block (14 oz) Extra-Firm Tofu: Think of it as a giant dog toy made of bean curd – and yes, it's way more delicious than it sounds (for you and your pup). Drain and press out any excess moisture – nobody likes a soggy scramble, not even a dog who just licked the floor.

- 1 Tablespoon Olive Oil: Because even healthy food needs a little lubrication.

- ½ Cup Chopped Onion: For that sniff-tastic goodness that'll have your pup cocking their head in confusion (and maybe drooling a little).

- ½ Cup Chopped Bell Pepper (Any Color!): Because colorful food is fun food, even for furry friends.

- ½ Cup Chopped Mushrooms: Cremini, shiitake, white button – your pup won't care, they'll just be happy it's not kibble again.

- ¼ Teaspoon Turmeric: A superfood for both humans and pups (with vet approval, of course).

- ¼ Teaspoon Ground Cumin: Because exotic spices are the new kibble on the block.

- Pinch of Black Pepper: A little kick for pups who like things interesting (but start small, some pups have delicate palates).

- ¼ Cup Water or Vegetable Broth: Because nobody likes a dry scramble, not even a dog who just rolled in the mud (although, they might not complain…).

Instructions:

The Great Tofu Transformation: Drain and press that tofu like you're trying to wring out a wet dishcloth. Then, crumble it into a bowl using your hands or a fork. Imagine you're making doggy-sized scrambled eggs – but way less messy (hopefully).

Sautéing for the Snoot-Enticingly Rank Mixed Goodness: Intensity up that olive oil in a skillet and throw in the slashed onion, chime pepper, and mushrooms. Sauté them for 5-7 minutes, or until they're delicate and marginally carmelized. Your dog's tail will wag like a metronome with the note "excited" as soon as you hear the delicious aromas wafting through the kitchen.

Spice Up That Scramble Life (But Not Too Much): Add the turmeric, cumin, and black pepper. Sauté for another minute, letting those spices release all their wonderful doggy-approved aromas. Be careful with the pepper though – some pups like things blander than yesterday's newspaper.

Tofu Joins the Pawty: Dump that crumbled tofu into the pan with the veggies and stir it all together. Cook for 3-4 minutes, stirring often, to heat the tofu through. Basically, you're turning it into yummy, dog-safe scrambled eggs.

Moisture Makes It Magnificent: Pour in that water or vegetable broth and stir it all up. Cook for another minute or two, letting the liquid get absorbed. You don't want a soupy mess, but you also don't want your pup choking on dry tofu bits.

Serving Suggestions:

Let the tofu scramble cool down a bit – you don't want your pup burning their tongue (unless they, you know, ate your favorite shoes again). Portion it out into bowls and serve. This recipe can be enjoyed on its own, or spooned over cooked brown rice or quinoa for a meal that'll leave your pup feeling like the top dog (because, let's face it, they are).

Flavorful Variations: Taking Your Tofu Scramble to the Next Level

The base recipe is a blank canvas, ready for your pup's inner Picasso to go wild! Here are some ideas to get you started:

- **The Hearty Hound Scramble:** Add ½ cup of cooked lentils or chopped cooked tempeh for a protein punch that'll leave your pup feeling like they could run a marathon (or at least chase the mailman for an extra block).

- **The Fire-Breathing Fury Scramble:** Feeling adventurous? Include a pinch of red pepper flakes (adjust based on your pup's spice tolerance) with the spices. Just remember, some pups like things spicy like a jalapeno popper, while others prefer bland like yesterday's kibble. Proceed with caution!

- **The Fresh Breath Frenzy Scramble:** For a flavor twist that'll make your pup's kisses a little less, well, "doggy," stir in a tablespoon of chopped fresh parsley or cilantro after cooking. Just be sure they don't eat the whole tablespoon – that much green might make them see squirrels everywhere.

Coconut Rice: The Sidekick That Steals the Show

This ain't your average doggy rice! Coconut rice is like a tropical vacation in a bowl, and it's the perfect accompaniment to your pup's tofu masterpiece.

Ingredients:

- 1 cup long-grain white rice (because sometimes basic is beautiful)

- 1 ½ cups unsweetened coconut milk (because a little coconutty goodness never hurt anyone... or any dog)

- 1 cup water (for hydration, because even doggy adventures require staying hydrated)

- ½ teaspoon salt (optional, consult your veterinarian about adding salt to your dog's food)

Instructions:

- The Incomparable Rice Gather Together: Consolidate every one of the fixings (rice, coconut milk, water, and perhaps some salt) in a pot. Increase the heat to medium and bring the mixture to a boil to bring the party to a boil. The fun begins here, when your dog will start doing zoomies around your ankles and the kitchen will be filled with the delicious aroma of coconut. Cool off At this point: When it bubbles, lessen the intensity to low, cover the dish, and stew for 18-20 minutes. You want the rice to be cooked through and absorb all of the liquid; in other words, you want rice perfection. Take the pan off the heat and fluff the rice with a fork after it has finished cooking. It's like making a fluffy, soft, and probably delicious dog cloud.

Serving Suggestions:

- Serve the coconut rice as a side dish next to the tofu scramble. Let your pup choose their culinary adventure – some like things separate, others prefer the combination.

- Feeling fancy? Spoon the tofu scramble over a bed of that fluffy coconut rice. Instant gourmet doggy dinner!

Tips From the Top Dog Chef:

- **Fresh is Best:** This recipe uses cooked ingredients, but consider giving your pup a side of steamed green beans or chopped broccoli for some extra vitamins and hydration. They might not love it, but a good doggy parent provides a balanced meal (and maybe a belly rub afterwards to make up for it).

- **Portion Patrol:** How much your pup eats depends on their size, age, and activity level. Talk to your vet about appropriate serving sizes for your furry friend.

- **Leftovers Aren't for Suckers:** Both the tofu scramble and coconut rice can be stored in separate airtight containers in the fridge for up to 3 days. Reheat gently before serving – nobody likes fridge-temperature food, not even a dog who stole your socks this morning (no judgment).

With a little creativity, the tofu scramble can be transformed from ordinary to extraordinary. So get out there, experiment with flavors, and create a meal that will have your pup howling

with delight!

Chapter 8

DELICIOUS AND FUNCTIONAL TREATS FOR TRAINING AND REWARDS

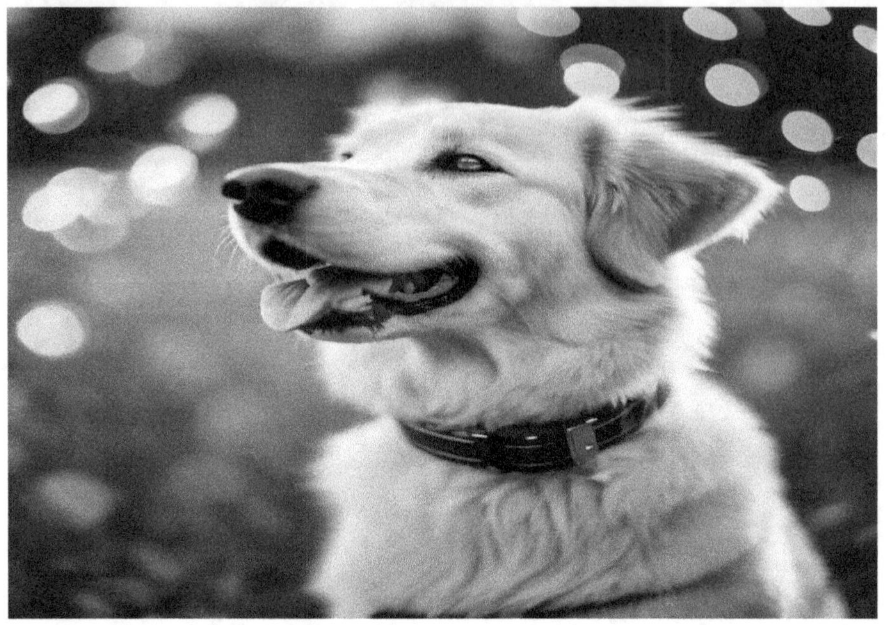

Baked Apple and Oat Bites

Turn Your Pup into a Snack-Craving Training Machine (But Not Really)

Tired of your dog acting like they haven't a single clue what "sit" means? Who are we kidding, they *totally* know what it means, they're just playing us for treats. Well, fret no more! This recipe is the ultimate bribe – er, I mean training tool –

that will have your furry friend begging to learn (or at least drool impressively).

Here's what you'll need to unleash your inner doggy treat baker:

- 1 cup rolled oats (because, hello, fiber for those zoomies)

- 1 cup unsweetened applesauce (like applesauce for yourself? Don't be greedy, share with your pup pal!)

- ½ cup grated apple (skin on, core removed – because nature's candy shouldn't be fussy)

- ¼ cup mashed banana (ripe – because who wants a grumpy, green banana treat?)

- 1 tablespoon ground flaxseed (mixed with 3 tablespoons of warm water to create a gel – it's like a super seed party in their mouth!)

- ½ teaspoon ground cinnamon (optional – some pups like it spicy, you do you)

Now, onto the fun part (besides watching your dog stuff their face):

1. **Preheat the Oven:** Crank that heat to 350°F (175°C) – imagine it as bribing your dog with a warm hug... in edible form. Line a baking sheet with parchment paper – 'cause cleaning baked-on banana is no picnic.

2. **Dry Ingredient Dance Party:** In a big bowl, throw together the rolled oats and cinnamon (if your dog's feeling fancy).

3. **Wet Ingredient Mashing Mayhem:** Grab another bowl and unleash your inner banana masher. Then, grate that apple like nobody's watching (or maybe your dog is, with increasing treat anticipation). Add the applesauce to the mashed banana and grated apple –

mush it all together until it's smooth like a puppy's belly.

4. **The Great Combine:** Pour the wet ingredients into the bowl with the dry ingredients. Don't forget the flaxseed gel – it's the glue that holds this delicious bribe... I mean training tool... together. Mix it all up until it's a sticky, glorious mess.

5. **Shaping the Rewards:** Now comes the fun part! Use a spoon or your hands (whichever your dog judges less) to scoop out giant spoonfuls of dough. Roll them into balls – think mini doggy meatballs. Place them on the baking sheet with some space between them so they don't become one giant apple oat monster.

6. **Bake Me to the Moon!:** Pop those treats in the oven for 15-20 minutes, or until they're firmish and starting to brown around the edges. Basically, until they look like they could bribe... er, train... any dog.

Tips:

Watch Those Chompers!

Baking time? More like barking time! These bite-sized treats are small, but they can burn faster than your pup can chase a squirrel. Keep your eye on them, or you might end up with hockey pucks instead of happy hour snacks.

Cool Your Jets (and Treats)

Hold your horses, Rover! These ain't fresh out of the oven lava bites. Let them cool completely before you unleash your furry friend on them. Nobody wants a burnt tongue, not even a fire hydrant-loving canine.

Stashing the Scooby Snacks

Leftovers? Don't worry, they won't go to waste (unlike that expensive chew toy you bought last week). Pop them in an airtight container at room temperature for a week. If your pup has serious self-control (doubtful), fridge them for two weeks, or freeze them for the ultimate "archaeology for kibble" challenge.

These Ain't Your Grandma's Cookies (But They're Still Delicious)

These treats are like tiny powerhouses of health! The oats are basically fiber highways, the apples are chock full of vitamins that might actually make your dog see straight (doubt it), and the flaxseed? Well, let's just say it's like doggy hairball medicine, but way tastier.

Spice Up Your Pup's Life (Without the Pepperoni)

Want to keep Fido's taste buds from getting bored? Here's where things get gourmet!

- **Sweet Potato Twist:** Swap out some apple for mashed sweet potato. Basically, it's like giving your dog a tiny orange surprise!

- **Berry Blast:** Add some blueberries or raspberries. Just make sure they're fresh or frozen, because nobody wants mystery moldy surprises.

- **Pumpkin Power:** Feeling festive? Replace some applesauce with pumpkin puree. Just don't add any pie filling, or you might be cleaning up a technicolor mess later.

With a little creativity, you can turn these treats into a smorgasbord of deliciousness that will have your dog rolling over (for more, please!). Remember, a happy pup is a quiet pup (unless there's a squirrel outside, then all bets are off).

Frozen Banana and Peanut Butter Popsicles

Is your pup looking more like a panting puddle than a playful pooch? Blame summer! But fear not, fellow doggo devotee, for we have the answer – Frozen Banana and Peanut Butter Popsicles!

These ain't your fancy fruit freezies. These are cool concoctions designed to keep your canine companion chillin' like a villain on a hot day.

Ingredients:

- 2 mushy bananas (the riper, the easier to blend – just like your brain after a day at the dog park)
- ½ cup of yogurt (plain or something fancy like pumpkin or banana – just make sure it's dog-safe, unlike your questionable fashion choices) (Optional)
- ¼ cup of peanut butter (creamy or chunky, but hold the xylitol – that's toxic to pups!) (Optional)
- Bonus Funfetti (Optional):

- ½ cup of chopped berries (blueberries, raspberries, strawberries – the redder the better, because apparently that's what makes them scream "summer!")

- ¼ cup of chopped sweet potato (because who doesn't love a surprise orange in their popsicle?)

- ¼ cup of mashed green beans (hey, don't knock it till you try it – they're good for your pup and might even add some extra "oomph" to their next zoomies!)

Instructions:

1. **Banana Blitz:** Blend those bad boys (the bananas, not the boys) until they're smoother than a puppy's belly. You can also mash them with a fork if you prefer a popsicle with a bit more... texture (like the fur tumbleweeds that collect under your couch).

2. **Mix-In Mayhem:** Feeling fancy? Throw in some yogurt or those bonus funfetti we mentioned. Just remember, moderation is key – you don't want your pup to turn into a walking yogurt parfait.

3. **Peanut Butter Power (Use Sparingly!):** Now listen up, peanut butter is a treat, not a popsicle base. So, resist the urge to go overboard and add a small dollop to each mold. You can drizzle it on top, swirl it in for a marbled masterpiece, or just plop it in – your pup won't judge your artistic skills (unlike that squirrel who keeps mocking you from the tree).

4. **The Big Freeze:** Pour the banana mixture (sans peanut butter) into your popsicle molds, leaving some room at the top – frozen things expand, you know? Then, pop those popsicle sticks in and shove the whole thing in the freezer for at least 4 hours, or until your pup starts begging like a champion.

Serving Suggestions (Because We All Know How Excited Pups Get):

- **Temper, Temper, Fido!** Don't unleash the frozen fury right away. Let the popsicle soften a bit so your dog can enjoy it without turning into a human popsicle-chomping machine (choking hazard alert!).

- **Operation: Popsicle Supervision** (Optional, but highly recommended for messy eaters): Like a toddler with a new ice cream cone, your pup might need some supervision to avoid a frozen-peanut-butter-banana war zone on your floor.

- **Leftover Popsicle Hacks:** Extra popsicles? Freeze them in an airtight container for later. Just remember, they're not collector's items – use them before they turn into archeological artifacts at the back of your freezer.

Top Tips to Avoid a Canine Catastrophe:

- **The Ripeness Report:** Bananas with more spots than a Dalmatian are your best bet. They're sweeter, smoother, and basically the rockstars of the banana world.

- **Mix-In Madness:** Feeling like a doggy Da Vinci? Get creative with different fruits and veggies (minus the pits and seeds – those are doggie no-nos). Just remember, some mix-ins might lead to... interesting colorful deposits in your backyard.

- **Fresh is Always Fetch:** Frozen is good, but fresh water is essential. Keep a bowl of H2O handy to keep your pup hydrated, because even popsicles can't replace a good ol' fashioned slurp.

- **Portion Patrol:** Treats are treats, not a doggy buffet. Especially when it comes to peanut butter. Talk to your vet about portion sizes to avoid a furry belly ache the size of a beach ball.

The Bottom Line:

These popsicles are the bomb (the good kind, not the kind that explodes in your freezer). They're easy to make, keep your pup cool, and might even provide a much-needed potassium boost (because let's face it, chasing squirrels doesn't exactly count as exercise). Just remember, safety first! Consult your vet if you have any questions, and avoid letting your dog become a frozen-treat-fueled projectile. Happy summer!

Crunchy Chickpea and Veggie Cookies

These bad boys are bursting with protein and fiber, thanks to the mighty chickpea and a whole garden of dog-safe veggies. Forget boring kibble, these are like tiny weightlifting sessions for your furry friend's insides (okay, maybe not that intense, but still good!).

Ingredients:

- 1 cup chickpea flour (basically ground-up chickpeas, because who has time for fancy names?)

- ½ cup rolled oats, pulverized into dust (think super fine oatmeal – like your patience after cleaning up the last "present" in the backyard)

- ½ cup cooked and mashed sweet potato (because who doesn't love a surprise orange in their cookie?)

- ¼ cup unsweetened applesauce (the healthy sweetener, unlike that suspicious puddle of "mystery goo" you found under the couch)

- ¼ cup chopped veggies of your dog's choice (carrots for the sight-challenged, green beans for the eco-conscious pup, broccoli florets for the tiny tree-munching dinosaurs?)

- 2 tablespoons olive oil (for a little extra oomph)

- 1 tablespoon chia seeds (optional, but they look fancy and might give your dog chia-tastic superpowers)

- Water (as needed, because sometimes things get a little dry... like your dog's enthusiasm for that squeaky toy you bought last week)

Instructions:

1. **Preheat the Oven to "Golden Brown":** Crank that oven to 350°F (or 175°C for our metrically minded friends). Line a baking sheet with parchment paper – nobody wants a sticky situation.

2. **The Great Flour Fusion:** In a big bowl, whisk together the chickpea flour, oat dust, and chia seeds (if you're feeling fancy).

3. **Sweet Potato Smash:** Grab another bowl and mash that sweet potato like it owes you money. Smooth is the name of the game.

4. **Mix it Up Like a Canine DJ:** Add the mashed sweet potato, applesauce, and olive oil to the dry ingredients.

Stir it all together until it becomes a thick dough. Think playdough, but way tastier (for dogs, at least). If it's drier than a dog park on a Tuesday afternoon, add a splash of water at a time until it becomes workable.

5. **Veggie Bonanza!** Now comes the fun part: Chop up those pup-approved veggies and toss them in the dough. Make sure they're evenly distributed – you don't want your doggo to become a green-bean-obsessed picky eater.

6. **Shaping Smackdown:** There are two ways to tackle this:

   ○ **Rolling and Cutting (for the Precise Pup):** Lightly flour a surface and roll out the dough to about ¼ inch thickness. Then, grab some cookie cutters and create fun shapes! Think paw prints, bones, or even tiny fire hydrants (because everyone loves a good fire hydrant, right?). If you don't have cookie cutters, a knife will do just fine – squares are totally in this season.

- ○ **Scooping and Shaping (for the Free-Spirited Pup):** Use a spoon or a cookie scoop to portion out the dough onto your baking sheet. Lick your fingers (just kidding... maybe) and gently pat the dough balls into flattened cookies.

7. **The Big Bake:** Pop those cookies in the oven for 15-20 minutes, or until they're golden brown and firm to the touch. Let them cool completely on the baking sheet before you unleash your furry friend on them.

Tips:

Experiment Like a Mad Scientist: Don't be afraid to sub out those veggies! Bell peppers, zucchini, even green peas (just don't tell your dog they're basically eating tiny green bouncy balls) are all fair game. Just remember, some veggies might lead to... interesting colorful surprises in your backyard later.

Fresh or Frozen? You Decide! Both fresh and frozen veggies work here. But for frozen veggies, thaw them completely and squeeze out any extra moisture. Nobody wants a soggy cookie, not even your dog (unless they're secretly a swamp monster disguised as a canine).

Storage Wars: The Cookie Edition Leftover cookies? Stash them in an airtight container at room temperature for a week, or shove them in the fridge for two weeks. If you're feeling like a super-prepared pup parent, freeze them for even longer storage.

These **Crunchy Chickpea and Veggie Cookies** are the perfect way to combine treat time with a little nutritional roulette. They're delicious, they're healthy-ish, and they might even keep your dog guessing about what veggie surprise awaits them in each bite. Just remember, consult your vet before making any major changes to your dog's diet, and maybe lay down some newspaper – you never know how your pup will react to these veggie treats!

Chapter 9

HOMEMADE SUPPLEMENTS AND REMEDIES FOR COMMON CANINE AILMENTS

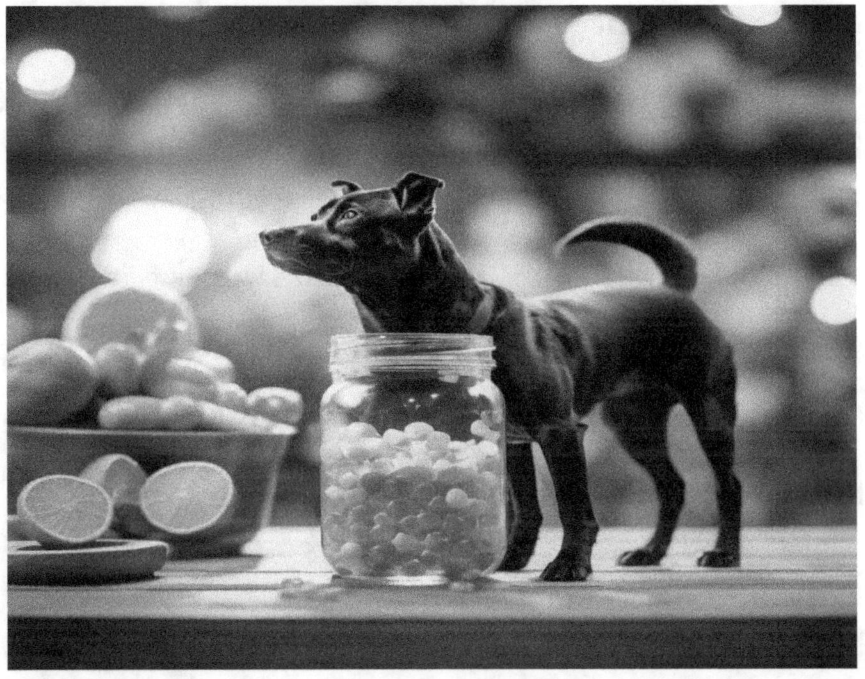

Soothing Probiotic Pumpkin Puree for Digestion

Does your dog's digestion resemble a malfunctioning washing machine on spin cycle? Loud noises, questionable smells, and a general sense of chaos? Fear not, fellow pet parent, for we have the answer – **Soothing Probiotic Pumpkin Puree!**

But First, a Science Lesson (Kind Of):

Imagine your dog's gut as a microscopic battleground. On one side, the good guys – tiny warriors called probiotics. On the other side, the bad guys – well, let's just say they cause some serious digestive distress. This pumpkin puree is basically a superhero serum for those good guys, helping them win the battle and keep your dog's tummy troubles at bay.

Here's the Superfood Breakdown:

- **Probiotics:** Think of them as microscopic cheerleaders, rallying the good gut bacteria to keep things running smoothly.

- **Pumpkin:** This orange wonder is basically fiber heaven. It bulks things up and gets everything moving in the right direction (if you catch my drift).

Ingredients:

- 1 cup of unsweetened canned pumpkin puree (not that pie filling stuff – that's like giving your dog dessert before dinner)

- 1 tablespoon of plain, unflavored yogurt (with live cultures, but hold the sprinkles!) (Optional)

- Warm water (as needed, because sometimes things get a little thick... like your dog's... well, you get it)

Instructions:

1. **The Great Pumpkin Puree and Yogurt Fusion:** In a bowl, combine the pumpkin puree and yogurt (if you're feeling fancy).

2. **Adjusting the Consistency:** If it looks like wallpaper paste, add a splash of warm water at a time until it's, well, not like wallpaper paste.

Serving Suggestions:

- Serve this magic potion on its own, or mix it in with your dog's regular food.

- Start small, especially if your pup is a picky eater (or has a sensitive tummy). You can gradually increase the amount as their digestive system adjusts.

- For best results, serve this concoction once or twice a day when your dog's stomach decides to declare war.

Disclaimer: This is not a magic cure-all. If your dog's tummy troubles persist, consult your vet. But with a little pumpkin power, you might just turn your gassy gremlin back into the happy hound you know and love.

Tips:

This ain't your grandma's pumpkin pie filling. We're talking fresh, fabulous pumpkin puree – the kind that won't give your pup a sugar rush or a bellyache. Think of it as a digestive Dougie – smooth moves guaranteed!

Probiotics: Choosing the Right Yogurt for Your Yogurt-Loving Yapper

Just like picking out a swimsuit, consult your vet for the paw-fect probiotic yogurt. Look for one that specifically mentions live and active cultures – basically, a yogurt party in your pup's tummy!

Monitor Your Marvelous Mutt:

This recipe is supposed to be a digestive dance party, but if your dog starts doing the Macarena instead (think uncontrollable... well, you get it), stop the music and call your vet.

Chamomile Tea: Nature's Chill Pill for Canine Chaos

Chamomile – it's like a tiny, daisy-shaped peace offering for your pup. People have been using it to unwind for ages, and maybe, just maybe, it can turn your furry friend into a mellow marshmallow.

Chamomile might be a natural doggy downer, helping them relax during those earsplitting thunderstorms or firework fiestas. Feeling anxious can wreak havoc on a dog's digestion. Chamomile might be able to help smooth things over down there. While some swear by chamomile tea for chilled-out pups, scientists are still scratching their heads about how well it actually works. Chamomile is generally safe in small amounts, but a chat with your vet is key before you turn your pup into a tea-guzzling fiend. They can help you figure out the right amount based on your dog's size, breed, and any other health issues. Chamomile tea is great for occasional anxiety, but for serious doggy drama, consult your vet for a proper diagnosis and treatment plan. Remember, this is just a helping paw. Consulting your vet is always the best way to ensure your doggo is happy and healthy!

How to Use Chamomile Tea for Dogs (Always consult your veterinarian before using):

Does your dog bounce off the walls like a furry pinball? Chamomile tea might be the answer to your prayers (and your sanity).

Brewing a Batch of Canine Chill:

1. **Steeping the Sleepy Stuff:** Toss 1-2 teaspoons of dried chamomile flowers into hot water for 5-10 minutes. Think of it like making a tea party for your pup, minus the fancy hats and cucumber sandwiches.

2. **Cool it Down, Woof Woof!:** Let that tea turn lukewarm before offering it to your pup. You wouldn't want to burn their little tongue!

3. **Start Small, Sherlock Bones:** Introduce a tiny amount (a teaspoon or two) to your dog's water bowl. See if they take to it like a duck to... well, water. Watch

for any allergic reactions or tummy troubles – we don't want a chamomile catastrophe!

Word to the Wise from the Vet:

- **Talk to Your Vet First:** If your dog seems to dig the chamomile and you want to make it a regular thing, chat with your vet about proper dosage and how often to serve it.

- **Chamomile: Not a Magic Potion:** This tea might help with occasional anxiety, but it's not a guaranteed fix. Consulting your vet is always the best way to tackle your dog's anxiety and keep them happy and healthy.

Remember, this is just a tail-wagging tip. Consulting your vet is always the best course of action for your furry friend!

Fresh Breath Parsley and Mint Dog Chews

Tired of your dog's breath making houseguests faint? Introducing Fresh Breath Parsley and Mint Dog Chews - the ultimate weapon in the war against canine halitosis (don't worry, we googled that one for you). These chews are so effective, you might even be able to get close enough to cuddle without needing a hazmat suit.

But wait, there's more! These chews aren't just breath fresheners, they're also a sneaky way to indulge your dog's natural chewing obsession. Think of it as a doggie pacifier, but instead of questionable rubber, it's made with all-natural ingredients that might even soothe their tummy troubles (hey, less mess for you to clean up, right?).

Now, onto the good stuff (bribery for your dog):

- **Ingredients:**

- 2 cups loosely packed fresh parsley leaves (washed and dried, because nobody wants swamp breath)
- ½ cup fresh mint leaves (washed and dried, same reason as above)
- 2 tablespoons unsalted, unsweetened applesauce (optional, but hey, it's like adding sprinkles to your dog's chew toy!)
- Water (as needed, because who wants a burnt chew toy? That's just depressing)

Instructions:

1. **Preheat the Oven:** Aim for low and slow, baby. Think of it as a relaxing spa day for your herbs, not a volcanic eruption. Around 175°F (80°C) should do the trick. Or, if you have one of those fancy dehydrator things, that works too.

2. **Herb Prep Time:** Wash those parsley and mint leaves like you mean it. You wouldn't want your dog to share breath fresher with a salad that fell in the dirt, would you? Stems? Up to you. Think of them as little handles for your dog to proudly display their new chew toy. Roughly chop the leaves - you're not aiming for gourmet presentation here, just get them nice and bite-sized.

3. **Shaping Up:**

   - **Spreading the Love:** Line a baking sheet with parchment paper and scatter those herbs like confetti at a doggy disco.

   - **Molding the Munchies (optional):** Want something a little more formed? Mix those chopped herbs with the applesauce (if you're feeling fancy) until you get a slightly sticky situation going. Don't worry, it's the good kind of sticky. Think Play-Doh for grown-up dogs. Mold the mixture into bite-sized shapes or spread it out on a lined baking sheet.

Drying the Chews:

Alright, here comes the exciting part (or maybe the really boring part, depending on how much you like watching paint dry): Drying these chews. Think of it as your dog's very own dental hygiene transformation sequence!

Oven Quest: Pop that baking sheet with your herbs (or molded masterpieces) into the preheated oven. But here's the twist - you gotta leave the door slightly open, like a sneaky teenager returning way past curfew. Prop a wooden spoon in the hinge to let all that doggy-breath-fighting moisture escape.

Dehydrator Dungeon: Got one of those fancy dehydrator things? Great! Follow its instructions like you're deciphering an ancient doggy scroll.

The Waiting Game (aka Netflix Time): Now comes the patience test. Bake (or dehydrate) that mixture for 2-4 hours, or until those leaves are drier than a pun about dry cleaners. Think of it as quality time with Netflix...while your dog waits impatiently for their breath-freshening prize.

How Do I Know They're Done? (The Crumble Test): Here's the science part: the chews are ready when the leaves turn into tiny green and white ninjas - completely brittle and ready to crumble at the touch. No more soggy, sad herbs allowed!

Cooling Down (Let's Not Get Burned!): Once those chews are cool enough to handle without scorching your fingers (because who needs doggy breath AND burnt fingertips?), take them out of the oven or dehydrator.

Treasure Chest Time (Storing the Goods): Now for the grand finale! Stash those chews in an airtight container, like a pirate hiding their treasure. Properly stored, these breath-blasting wonders can last up to a week.

Serving Up a Breath of Fresh Air: Now, the moment you've both been waiting for! Give your dog one or two of these Fresh Breath Parsley and Mint Dog Chews, but watch them like a hawk. We don't want any choking hazards, just minty-fresh chomping.

Important Side Note (Because We Don't Want Your Dog to Sue Us): Remember, these chews are like a doggy breath mint, not a magic shield. Brushing your pup's teeth regularly and scheduling vet cleanings are still super important for their pearly whites.

So there you have it! Fresh Breath Parsley and Mint Dog Chews - a simple (and hopefully not too boring) way to fight doggy halitosis and keep your furry friend's smile sparkling (well, maybe not sparkling, but definitely less like a dumpster fire).

Chapter 10

MONITORING YOUR DOG'S HEALTH ON A VEGAN DIET

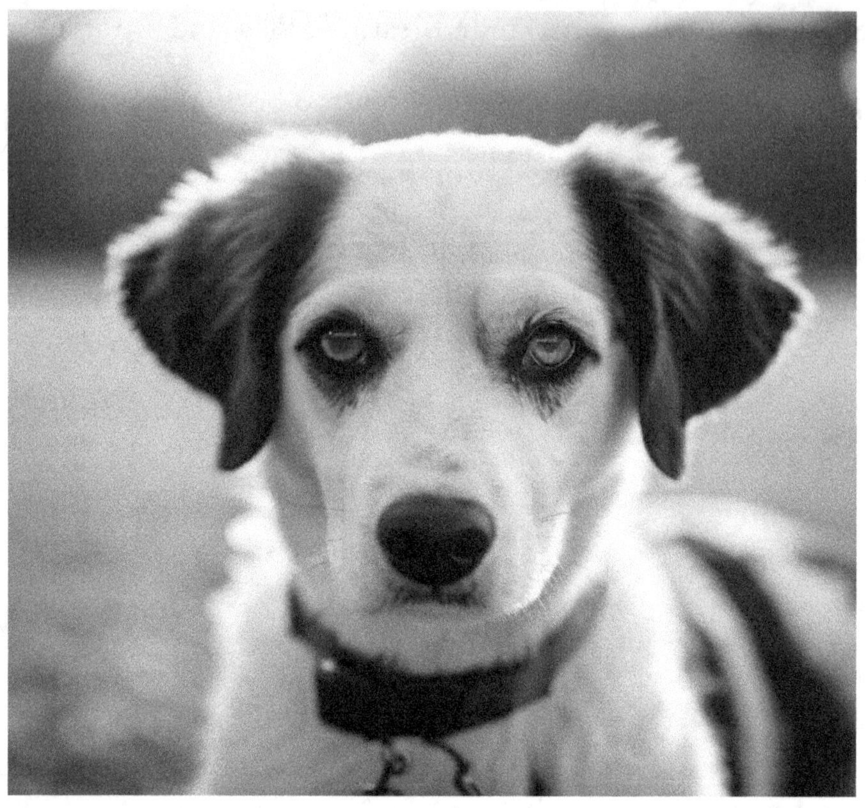

Recognizing Signs of Nutritional Deficiencies

So, you've decided to turn your pup into a plant-powered pal. Awesome! But before your dog becomes the hippest hound at the park, we gotta make sure their new nosh isn't leaving them feeling ruff.

This chapter is basically a doggy detective guide to sniffing out signs that your vegan diet might be missing some key ingredients. Think of it like canine CSI: Kibble Scene Investigation.

Important Disclaimer: We're here for laughs, not diagnoses. If your furball seems off, get them to a vet, stat! They're the real heroes with the stethoscopes.

Meat-Free Meals, Meat-FULL Needs:

It has been discovered that even these endearing scavengers necessitate a diet that is well-rounded in nature. In contrast to their capricious feline counterparts who are obligate carnivores, dogs are classified as omnivores. They have the ability to consume both flora and fauna. However, it is imperative to acknowledge that their vegetarian meals require a substantial level of empirical scrutiny in order to guarantee that all nutritional requirements are adequately met. We're talking protein power for those playful pounces, healthy fats for a fur that shines brighter than a disco ball, and just the right amount of carbs for zoomies that would make a cheetah jealous. So, how do you know if your pup's plant-based plate is packing the punch it needs? Well, their body might start throwing some not-so-subtle hints. We're talking a dull coat drier than a day-old bagel, or energy levels that would make a sloth say, "Whoa, slow down there, champ!"

Don't worry, we'll delve into those signs deeper than a dachshund digging for treats. But remember, this isn't a substitute for a vet visit. They're the ultimate doggy dietary detectives!

Signs of Potential Nutritional Deficiencies:

Indubitably, the act of hastily consuming kale chips may indeed be deemed fashionable within the sphere of contemporary human hipsters, but one must ponder whether the adoption of a vegan diet is suited for one's beloved quadruped companion. Although a meticulously crafted plant-based sustenance can offer an abundance of essential nutrients for your canine companion, the repercussions of improper implementation could be dire. Hence, it is imperative to ascertain whether your furry friend's spiritual inclinations towards a dietary regimen devoid of animal products are yielding unfavorable physical manifestations.

Your Dog's Gone From Fabio to Furry Scruffball: Dry, itchy skin, shedding like a blizzard, and a coat duller than a week-old dishrag? Your dog might be missing out on essential fatty acids or certain vitamins. Time to ditch the hemp seed and load up on the lentil stew!

Digestive Disaster Zone: Vomiting, the runs, or constipation acting like a party guest who just won't leave? It could be a lack of fiber or trouble digesting all that plant-based protein. Maybe lay off the tofu scrambles for a bit, Fido.

The Zoomies Have Zoomed Away: Lethargy, fatigue, or a total lack of enthusiasm for fetch? This could mean your canine companion isn't getting enough calories or is missing key nutrients to keep their energy levels up. Put down the kombucha and pick up the kibble, stat!

Where'd All the Junk in the Trunk Go?: Weight loss despite chowing down like a champion eater? It might be a protein deficiency. Maybe swap out some lentil loaf for some lentil loaf with a side of... you guessed it, meat!

Night Blindness? More Like No Sight!: If your dog is bumping into walls more than usual, it could be a sign of vitamin A deficiency. Carrots, anyone?

And now for the not-so-secret secret: Regular vet checkups are as important for your dog as that monthly mani-pedi is for you. Think of it like taking your car in for an oil change – gotta keep that engine purring (or barking) smoothly!

Here's why those vet visits are pawsome:

Veterinarians possess the ability to detect incipient health issues prior to their escalation into significantly unpleasant olfactory manifestations. The timely identification of such concerns enables prompt medical intervention, yielding advantageous outcomes for all parties involved, most notably one's financial resources. Routine assessments address a helpful event to regulate to one's canine sidekick the full supplement of preventive clinical consideration they require, similar to inoculations, bug and tick stuff (since no one loves those frightening little creatures!), and dental cleanings (new pup breath, anybody?). The vet can survey your canine's weight, by and large body, fur circumstance, and general state of mind during an exam. This analyst work distinguishes any tricky medical problems that may brew.

Your Dog is Officially Old: How to Not Freak Out (and Maybe Even Enjoy It?)

Thus, your canine's formally a granddad (or grandmother!) of the world of dogs. Congrats! However, a whole new set of requirements for medical care come along with the distinctive grey muzzle and wisdom-filled eyes—or maybe just cataracts. This is the way to explore those vet visits without feeling like you're finishing up interminable pup tax documents.

Why Regular Checkups Become Super Important Now:

Think of your dog as a classic car. They may not be quite the spry pup they once were, and that engine needs a little more tinkering to keep it purring (or barking) happily. Regular checkups are like taking your furry friend to the mechanic – gotta make sure everything is running smoothly and catch any gremlins before they cause a major breakdown.

Becoming BFFs with Your Vet (Because Emergencies Happen):

The more your vet knows about your dog, the better! Regular checkups are like building a best-friendship with your veterinarian. This way, your veterinarian won't have to do any detective work if your dog ever experiences an unanticipated health complication. It resembles having a pup clinical attendant - they know your little guy's eccentricities and can give them the most potential customized care. How frequently ought to you take your dog to the vet? (Sit back and relax, they subtly partake in the vehicle ride): Very much like the way that a few people need the rec center more than others, how frequently your canine necessities an exam relies upon their age, breed, wellbeing, and in general way of life. Here is a super-improved on guide: Pups: Consider them little, charming clinical secrets. They need continuous exams, similar to like clockwork until they're around a half year old. All of their vaccinations are also most effective at this time. Grown-up Canines (Ages 1-7): Solid grown-up canines can for the most part drift by with yearly tests. Senior Canines (7+ Years Old): These recognized honorable men (and noble women) could require exams at regular intervals or considerably on a more regular basis, contingent upon their wellbeing. Keep in mind, this is only a general guide. Continuously counsel your veterinarian to sort out the ideal exam plan for your particular canine sidekick.

What Happens During a Checkup? It's Not All Prodding and Poking (Okay, Maybe a Little):

A customary veterinary examination can be likened to an indulgent pampering session for a dog, accompanied by medical procedures. The anticipated routine during such appointments is as follows:

Engaging in Dialogue about Prior Events: The veterinarian will inquire about the comprehensive medical background of your canine companion, including details concerning previous maladies, surgical interventions, and ongoing medication regimens. Essentially, this phase represents an opportunity for sharing pertinent information akin to canine discourse.

The Enormous Once-Finished: The vet will give your canine a full-body examination, really taking a look at their eyes, ears, teeth, and in the middle between. Consider it a criminal investigator searching for pieces of information (of good wellbeing, ideally!). The Weigh-In: Your canine will jump on the scale to check whether their weight is in the sound zone for their variety and size. However, no strain to squeeze into a pup two-piece! Shots Up! (Perhaps): The vet will check whether your canine necessities any inoculations and try them out (with a yummy treat subsequently, obviously!). Parasite Watch: Vets are like knights doing combating the malevolent bugs and ticks! They'll talk about parasite avoidance choices and suggest the best weapons (prescription or deterrents) to keep those frightening little animals under control.

Your Canine's Exam: More Fun Than a Letter box Brimming with Squirrels! Thus, your canine's vet visit is approaching. Try not to picture miserable little dog eyes and cries of gloom. This can be an awe-inspiring experience, loaded up with much more fun than attempting to clear up for the postal worker why your valued bite toy has a place there! Chow Time, Fido Release: Your vet can be your canine's very own food master! They'll dole out all the soil (the great kind, we guarantee) on the right nourishment for your little guy's age, breed, and action level. Consider it a customized pup menu - no more asking for chomps of your kale salad (they presumably wouldn't care for it in any case). Don't ask! No Inquiry is Excessively Odd: Does your sleeping dog speak Dachshund? They might suddenly become obsessed with licking the rug in the living room. This is your opportunity to release a flood of inquiries on the vet. They're essentially pup clairvoyants, prepared to interpret your shaggy companion's secretive ways of behaving.

Regular Checkups: An Investment in Those Happy Tail Wags:

Ensuring regular veterinary examinations for your canine companion is akin to investing in the Happiness Canine Reserve. The primary objective is to safeguard their sustained well-being and contentment. Early identification of potential maladies in dogs, administering preventive measures to maintain their optimal health, and cultivating a harmonious relationship with their veterinarian – epitomizes the quintessential standard of conscientious pet guardianship, particularly emblematic in the Golden Retriever breed. Essentially, by adhering to these practices, one affords their furry friend the greatest opportunity for a protracted existence characterized by affectionate caresses, delectable treats, and ceaseless sessions of retrieving objects (for who can resist the captivating allure of those endearing, canine optics?).

Bloodwork: Decoding the Doggy Code:

The process of conducting bloodwork and tests can be likened to a sophisticated and advanced detective kit employed by the veterinary professional. These diagnostic tools are utilized to meticulously evaluate the comprehensive well-being of your canine companion, identify and address any underlying issues proactively before they escalate into severe complications, and monitor the progression of any pre-existing medical conditions with a watchful eye.

Catching the Bad Guys Early:

Bloodwork can be a lifesaver, uncovering hidden health issues before they cause any trouble. Think of it as catching the doggy villain before they can unleash their reign of chaos (like, say, the Great Sock-Stealing Caper of 2024). Early detection means early treatment, which usually leads to a happier, healthier pup.

Keeping an Eye on Those Pre-Existing Conditions:

Does your dog have a bit of a medical history? Bloodwork and tests can be like a trusty sidekick, helping your vet monitor how well their treatment is working and keeping an eye on any changes in their condition.

Surgical Checkup: Making Sure Your Pup is Ready for Action!:

Hematological analysis serves as a preparatory assessment akin to a pre-operational debriefing for canines undergoing surgical procedures. This analysis enables the veterinarian to ascertain the animal's fitness to withstand both anesthesia and the surgical intervention itself. Essentially, it is aimed at ensuring that your canine companion is adequately prepared to endure the inevitable discomfort associated with post-operative attire, maintaining their composure and decorum throughout. Genetic predispositions in dog breeds play a pivotal role in determining vulnerabilities to specific health conditions. Hematological tests and demonstrative evaluations act as a vital device in disentangling these hereditary susceptibilities, offering bits of knowledge to the veterinarian with respect to any potential variety explicit medical problems at a beginning phase. Mindfulness and readiness are fundamental parts in guaranteeing the prosperity and life span of our canine mates. Unraveling Your Pet's Clinical Secrets: An Aide That Won't Make You Bark With Disarray Thus, your vet referenced some bloodwork and tests for your little guy. Don't worry, this isn't a doggy version of the SATs! This guide will help you decipher those fancy medical terms and understand what's going on under your furry friend's fur.

Bloodwork: Like CSI for Canine Clues

Hematological analysis is essentially akin to investigative work for the veterinarian. They will be examining various diagnostic tests, each serving as a minuscule magnifying instrument to obtain a clearer understanding of the canine's well-being. The principal assessments include:

1. The Full Blood Count (FBC): This serves as a fundamental analysis of the canine's blood. It assesses the red blood cells (responsible for oxygen transportation), white blood cells (the body's defense mechanism), platelets (involved in blood clotting), and hemoglobin (the oxygen-carrying component). Essentially, this examination enables the veterinarian to determine whether the dog's immune system is actively responding, if blood coagulation is functioning properly, and if the overall health status is commendable.

2. The Serum Chemistry Panel: Think of this as a comprehensive physical examination for the canine. Electrolytes (similar to sports drinks for dogs), liver enzymes (an indicator of the liver's health), kidney parameters (crucial for waste elimination), protein levels (essential for bodily functions), and blood glucose (to determine the dog's activity level) are all examined in this evaluation. This analysis helps determine whether the dog is living a sedentary or active lifestyle. 3. Urinalysis: This evaluation is somewhat direct. The canine gives an example, and the veterinarian inspects it to distinguish possible signs of urinary lot diseases, bladder stones, kidney inconveniences, or diabetes. Luckily, this errand is solely attempted by the veterinary expert. X-Beam Vision: Seeing Past the Fur For your veterinarian, X-rays are like a superhero dog's vision. They can see through fur and get a brief look at bones, joints, and, surprisingly, inward organs. This can assist in the identification of fractures (ugh!), tumors (ugh!), and other hidden problems.

Ultrasound: A Deep Dive into the Doggy Depths

Ultrasound is like an underwater adventure for your vet, but instead of coral reefs, they're exploring your dog's soft tissues like organs. This can be helpful in finding certain cancers, diagnosing reproductive problems, and seeing what's going on deep down inside your pup.

Choosing the Right Tests: Not a One-Size-Fits-All Deal

So, which tests does your dog really need? There's no one-size-fits-all answer here. Here's a paw-print to consider:

Age: Puppies and senior pups might need more checkups and bloodwork due to their growing or aging bodies. Think of it as keeping a close eye on your little furball during their early years and giving extra TLC to your distinguished gentleman (or gentlewoman) in their golden years.

Breed: Some breeds are more prone to certain health problems. Just like some humans are more likely to be lactose intolerant than others, some breeds might need specific tests to catch potential issues early on.

Signs: In instances where your canine companion is exhibiting aberrant behaviors such as increased episodes of vomiting or incidents of inappropriate elimination within the household, diagnostic procedures such as bloodwork and specialized tests can facilitate in pinpointing the underlying cause of these canine transgressions. Because they have a comprehensive understanding of your dog's overall well-being and medical history, your veterinarian's advice is invaluable in such situations. They will tailor their diagnostic evaluation recommendations to your beloved pet's particular health status and history. It is advisable to place trust in the expertise of these skilled professionals, for they hold the title of being equivalent to masterful practitioners in the realm of canine medicine.

Cost Considerations: Keeping it Woof-fordable

Bloodwork and tests can vary in price depending on the type of test, location, and vet. It is advisable to engage in deliberate conversation regarding the expenses associated with veterinary care prior to proceeding with any treatments. Certain pet insurance policies may even provide coverage for specific medical tests; therefore, it is advisable to explore these options if financial concerns are at the forefront of one's mind.

It is essential to acknowledge that the timely identification of any potential health issues is imperative in safeguarding the well-being and contentment of one's canine companion. By collaborating closely with a qualified veterinarian and acquiring a comprehensive understanding of the diagnostic procedures available, pet owners can pave the way for a prolonged and fulfilling life for their beloved furry companions. This may involve the provision of ample belly rubs, engaging in countless games of fetch, and perhaps even offering an extra treat or two for demonstrating exemplary behavior as a loyal and cherished member of the household.

Cracking the Code with Your Vet: No Need to Speak Dog Latin Here!

So, the vet mentioned some bloodwork and tests for your pup. Don't break out the doggy phrasebook just yet! This is where you and your vet have a heart-to-heart (or should we say, tail-wag to stethoscope?) about what's going on with your furry friend.

Spill the Kibble: Sharing Your Dog's Medical History

Think of this as doggy story time. Please ensure to provide comprehensive and detailed information concerning your canine companion's health background, including previous medical conditions and peculiar behavioral patterns they may exhibit (such as a sudden proclivity for licking household rugs). The more information you uncover, the more actually your veterinarian will actually want to survey potential medical problems. Shooting for the Right End goal: Your Interests and Questions Is your canine dozing more than expected? Perhaps they appear to be somewhat less keen on pursuing squirrels.

Presently's your opportunity to release a flood of inquiries on your vet. They're essentially pup mystics, prepared to translate your little guy's strange ways of behaving and address any concerns you have.

Bloodwork and Tests: Worth Their Weight in Milk-Bones

Bloodwork and tests could sound frightening, yet they're really similar to very cool instruments for your vet. These analytic tests help in the early discovery of potential medical problems for your pet, ultimately preventing more serious complications. Timely identification plays a crucial role in ensuring the overall well-being and happiness of your dog.

Collaboration with Your Veterinarian: Leveraging the Strength of Teamwork!

Consider yourself and your veterinarian as an effective partnership dedicated to your dog's health. Through correspondence, shared conversations with respect to your pet's prosperity, and an appreciation for the worth of indicative tests, you can mutually decide the most fitting consideration intend to keep up with your canine's ideal wellbeing. It is essential to stress that this procedure is simple and transparent. By engaging in honest conversations with your veterinarian, you can guarantee that your furry companion receives the necessary support for a long and healthy life, filled with love, playtime, and occasional treats for their obedience and loyalty.

Chapter 11

BUILDING A STRONG BOND WITH

YOUR VEGAN CANINE COMPANION

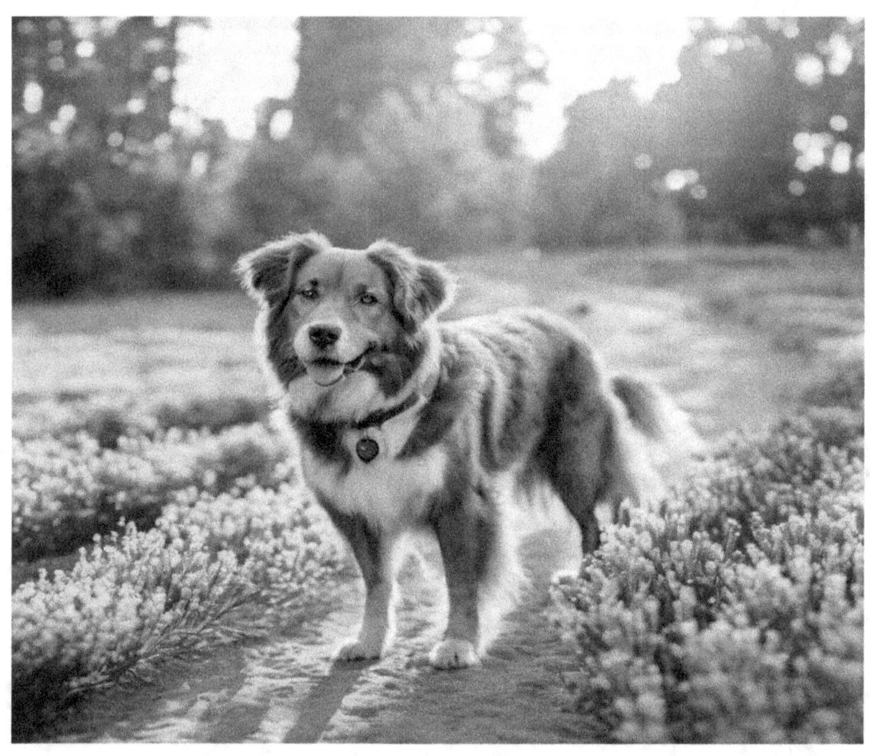

Exercise and Activity for a Healthy Lifestyle

Listen up, pawsome pet parents! Exercise ain't just for fancy hot dog-eaters, your vegan pup needs to get their wiggle on too! Think of it like this: exercise is like the zoomies button for your doggo, but way better behaved (and less likely to involve furniture redecoration).

Here's the lowdown on why getting your plant-powered pup moving is a tail-wagging good idea:

Burning the Treat Pouch: Just like their omnivorous cousins, vegan dogs need exercise to keep that beach bod in tip-top shape. Those extra veggie nuggets gotta go somewhere, right? Nobody wants a chunky monkey (unless it's a peanut butter kind!).

Muscles of Steel (Well, Tofu): Exercise helps build muscles, which makes your dog a superhero in their own right! Think about it - more muscle means better zooming, fetching, and squirrel chasing abilities. Basically, they'll be the Usain Bolt of the dog park (minus the fancy shoes).

Brain Power on High: Dogs are natural-born busybodies. Exercise keeps their minds sharp and prevents them from becoming bored out of their gourds (which, let's face it, can lead to some serious shoe-chewing incidents). A tired pup is a happy pup, and a happy pup means less chance of them turning your favorite slippers into chew toys.

BFF Fur-of all time: Exercise is a fabulous method for holding with your canine. Consider it a monster round of get for your fellowship! Additionally, you can train them with tasty treats during all of their playtime (because, let's face it, who can resist those puppy dog eyes?). Now, the Dos and Don'ts of Vegan Doggo Exercise: Steady minded individuals will win in the end: In the event that your canine is a habitual slouch convert, don't anticipate that they should go from zero to legend short-term. Begin with short strolls and bit by bit increment the force and span to keep away from any pulled hamstrings (or, you know, pulled tails). Hydration Station:

Water is key for all competitors, even the shaggy kind. Ensure your canine approaches a lot of H2O previously, during, and after their activity experiences. Refueling after a workout: Imagine your dog as a tiny vegan bodybuilder. After a decent exercise, they could require a little protein support. Discuss a post-exercise snack made especially for active dogs with your veterinarian. In any case, recollect, skirt the twofold cheeseburger (they're not a feline!). Pay attention to Your Little guy: Very much like people, canines have their cutoff points. Focus on your shaggy companion's energy levels and change action as needs be. On hot days, perhaps trade the stroll for some indoor recess. No one needs a crapped little guy, particularly in the singing sun. So that's it! Practice is a phenomenal method for keeping your veggie lover canine cheerful, solid, and prepared to vanquish the world (or if nothing else the neighborhood canine park). Keep in mind, a tiny amount arranging and a few fun exercises make a huge difference in guaranteeing your plant-controlled little guy carries on with their best life! Fun Exercises for Yourself as well as Your Veggie lover Canine: Okay, it's time to get those veggie-fueled paws pumping instead of taking naps on kibble! Here's the way things are looking: practice for your veggie lover canine isn't just about consuming off treat-instigated zoomies, it's an amazing experience for both of you. Think of yourselves as Lewis and Bark (get it?) as they explore the great outdoors—or, depending on the weather, your living room. Prepared to release your inward pack pioneer? Lock in for some tail-swaying fun: **Climbing with Bounces:** Hit the paths! Outside air, work out, and perhaps a squirrel experience (simply don't fault us in the event that your canine neglects they're on a vegetarian diet). Additionally, their super sniffer stays sharp from all the sniffing. The **Canine Kayak Club:** Does your canine cherish a decent sprinkle? Swimming is an incredible low-influence exercise that will make them paddle like a master (simply less the genuine oar... paws turn out great). Fetch? More Like Incredible Recovery Journey!: Bring and frisbee are works of art which is as it should be. Who doesn't cherish pursuing a flying item? Only be ready for an intermittent "fella, where'd it go?" second when your canine gets excessively into the chase (fault the kale for that careful attention!). **Dexterity:** From Habitual slouch to Ninja Fighter: Deftness courses resemble pup deterrent courses, ideal for keeping your little guy intellectually and actually invigorated. Simply envision the gloating freedoms at the canine park: "Goodness definitely, my canine absolutely scales that wall... on a vegetarian diet!"

Sniffari! Connect with the Super Sniffer: Recollect those treat-concealing games from your life as a youngster? Ends up, canines love them as well! Connect with their astounding feeling of smell by concealing kibble (veggie lover kibble, obviously!) around the house or yard. It resembles an implicit expedition for your fuzzy companion. Canine Olympics Anybody?: Feeling serious? If your dog secretly wants to be a mermaid—with fur—you should look into dog sports like obedience, rally, and even dock diving. It's a pleasant method for preparing, work out, and perhaps win a blue lace (which you can thoroughly casing and hold tight the refrigerator... close to the slobber commendable image of your little guy mid-air). Yet, pause, there's something else! Stormy days got you down? stuck inside with a zoomies case? Don't sweat it! Puzzle toys, intelligent feeders, and, surprisingly, short instructional courses can keep your little guy involved and intellectually invigorated. Keep in mind, the key is to find exercises you BOTH appreciate. A blissful canine is a sound canine, and a solid canine is a canine prepared to overcome the world (or if nothing else the local fire hydrant). By integrating these pleasant exercises into your daily practice, you'll make an enduring bond with your fuzzy companion and guarantee they carry on with a life that is however sound as it could be diverting. Why mental stimulation is so important: See, we as a whole realize practice is significant. But let's face it: your dog sometimes stares at the wall so intently that you wonder if they're thinking about life's meaning or just plotting your demise with chew toys. That is where mental excitement comes in, people. It resembles mind vigorous exercise for your shaggy companion, and here's the reason they need it:

Weariness Busters: An exhausted canine is a horrendous canine. Think destroyed furnishings, uncovered gardens, and an ensemble of barks that would humiliate Pavarotti. Mental excitement gives your canine a source for their energy and holds their little dark matter back from going to mush. Know it all College: Standard mental difficulties resemble pup Sudoku. They improve your dog's memory, ability to solve problems, and overall intelligence. This is particularly significant for senior canines, who could somehow forget where they concealed their valued sock assortment (or perhaps that is only mine?). **Holding Pals:** Instructional meetings and intuitive games are your opportunity to interface with your canine and tell them, "Hello, you're not only a slobber distributor!" Besides, giving them recognition and treats is a dependable method for turning into their generally most loved human (sorry, postal worker).

Turning Your Dopey Canine into a Doge-torate Holder: Positive Reinforcement Training

Forget yelling and yanking on leashes. Positive reinforcement training is the key to a happy, well-behaved dog (and a slightly saner you). Here's the lowdown:

- **Treat Time!:** Did your dog finally sit on command without looking like they're about to fall over? Treat time! Did they resist the urge to scarf down your entire shoe collection? More treat time! Positive reinforcement is all about rewarding good behavior, making your doggo think learning new tricks is the best thing since belly rubs.

Short and Sweet Sessions: Nobody likes a nag. Keep training sessions short and positive, like 5-10 minutes a few times a day. Think of it as quality time, not doggy boot camp.

- **Patience is a Virtue (Especially with Drool Monsters):** Learning takes time, so be patient with your pup. Repeat commands consistently, and don't get discouraged if they don't become Einstein overnight.

- **Fun is the Situation:** Preparing ought to be charming for both of you! Utilize a fun loving tone, consolidate games and exercises, and perhaps wear an entertaining cap to keep things fascinating. Who knows, your canine could try and show you a stunt or two (like how to shake a floppy-eared beret immaculately).

- **Mental Excitement Exercises for Veggie lover Canines:** Indeed, your canine may be shaking a savagery free way of life, yet that doesn't mean their cerebrum should be on a kale chip break! This is the way to keep your vegetarian little guy intellectually invigorated without falling back on dubious looking "secret meat" treats:

- **Think of these as doggy Rubik's Cubes for dinnertime:** food puzzles and interactive feeders. Top them off with vegetarian kibble or treats and watch your shaggy companion become a kibble-unearthing champion. Only be ready for the chance of a slobber shrouded floor simultaneously (hello, mental effort is parched work!).

- **Scent Work Games:** Make your dog feel like a truffle pig by hiding toys or treats made of vegan ingredients around the house. This takes advantage of their regular sniffer abilities and keeps their cerebrum speculating, all while fulfilling their base desire to track down covered treasure (ideally not your vehicle keys). Interesting Treats: Showing your canine new deceives is an oldie but a goodie for yourself and a psychological exercise for them. Think "sit," "shake," or "play dead" (with dramatic groans getting extra points!). Reward them with vegetarian treats, cleaved up veggies, or perhaps a minuscule cut of that entirely ready banana you've been peering toward (sharing is mindful, right?).

- **Doggy Da Vincis:** Ready to get creative? Prepare your own snuffle mats or find the stowaway toys utilizing reused materials and, obviously, vegetarian treats. It's like upcycling for your dog's mental health! Frozen Fun: Transform nibble time into a psychological long distance race! Freeze some vegetarian stock or yogurt (twofold check with your vet for safe choices) in a Kong toy or lick mat. Your canine will be cheerfully involved for a very long time, licking and moving that delicious treat into their holding up mouth.

- **Bite on This (Yet Make it Vegetarian):** Biting is a pup distraction for an explanation - it eases weariness and keeps their brains dynamic. Give an assortment of bite toys produced using safe, plant-based materials like hemp or reused plastic. Who needs rawhide when you can have a hempy bone that is great for the planet and your little guy's chompers? Keep in mind, the key is to find exercises your canine partakes in that get their brainwaves humming. By consolidating these thoughts, you can keep your vegetarian canine intellectually sharp, keep fatigue from transforming them into a slobber beast, and fortify your bond through the force of encouraging feedback preparing (and perhaps a couple of taken banana nibbles).

Additional Tips:

Can we just be real, your canine isn't precisely eager for a delicious steak. However, dread not, individual veggie pet parent! Your guide to creating a drool-free, tail-wagging utopia for your plant-powered dog can be found in this chapter. Let's face it: a happy dog is much less likely to chew your Birkenstocks or, er, impersonate a furry Roomba on your throw rug.

- **Figuring out Your Veggie lover Canine Companion:** These vegetarian pups, like their meat-loving relatives, have some fundamental requirements that are more important than their next kale chip.

- **Love and Consideration (Since Even Tofu Needs Cuddles):** Give your canine warmth! Nestles, recess, and encouraging feedback are like daylight for their shaggy little spirits. Simply try not to cover them - they actually need some space to breathe (and perhaps an opportunity to escape for a decent ear scratch behind the sofa).

- **Mental Feeling (Weariness Busters for the Without budweiser Mind):** Recall that time you abandoned your canine for five minutes and returned to a scene of "innovative deconstruction" including your number one toss pad? No doubt, mental feeling is critical.

- **For a fun game of "Sniff and Seek:** Edamame Edition," think interactive toys, veggie-filled puzzle feeders, or kibble hidden around the house.

- **Actual Activity (Get Those Legs Pumpin', However Hold the Milk-Bone):** Strolls, bring (with an out of control carrot toy, maybe?), or investigating new paths - keep your canine moving! Not exclusively will it assist them with remaining trim areas of strength for and, it'll likewise wear them out for a nap that doesn't include your newly washed clothing heap.

- **Safety and Security (Because a Happy Home Is a Fortress, Especially from Rogue Vacuum Cleaners):** Provide a comfortable bed (bonus points for organic, hemp-filled cushions!) and follow routines. Your dog will feel safe and secure in their tofu-tastic domain if you are consistent, and consistency is your friend.

- **Socialization (Making Friends Who Don't Care About Your Dog's Diet):** Going to a supervised dog park or dog daycare is a great way for your dog to meet other dogs and friendly people. Simply recollect, some park puppies may be a little confounded by the absence of bacon treats, so watch out for any "incidental" food trades. Keep in mind that you can create a haven for your plant-powered dog with a little imagination and the help of these helpful tips. All things considered, a blissful, balanced veggie lover canine is way less inclined to organize a tofu-filled unrest in your front room.

Tailoring the Environment for a Vegan Dog:

Without a doubt, all canines hunger for gut rubs and ear scratches, however our veggie lover pals have some specialty needs as well. Here is the lowdown on keeping your mercilessness free canine sidekick cheerful:

- **Chow Time:** Trench the kibble with secret meat bits and select connoisseur veggie lover canine food created by vet nutritionists who (ideally) don't wear sterile garments made of imperiled rhinos. Skip individuals food scraps - those veggie burgers are for you, not Fido. He might get gas attacks from strange spices that could clear a room (and not in a good way).
- **Chew on This (But Not That!):** Supply a smorgasbord of safe, chew-tastic toys made from hemp

(because who doesn't love a good buzz?), recycled plastic (because saving the planet is pawsome!), or durable rubber (because even vegan dogs gotta gnaw on something). This keeps them from using your favorite throw pillows as dental floss.

- **Training Treats? Hold the Tofu Steaks!**

Positive reinforcement training is key for these veggie pups. Building trust is extra important since they might be suspicious of you after all those "chicken" flavored treats turned out to be lentils in disguise.

- **Cultivating a Kaleidoscope of Canine Comfort:**

Quality Time: Snuggle sessions and playtime are mandatory! Fetch in the park, go for long walks (because chasing squirrels is a primal instinct, even for the tofu-loving set), or just sprawl on the couch together – just don't make them watch documentaries about the evils of the meat industry.

- **Speak Delicately and hold a Major Carrot:** Keep your voice quiet and delicate - hollering is so last season, furthermore, it could make them believe you're a military trainer attempting to transform them into a meat-eating machine.

- **Routine is Top dog (or Sovereign):** Set steady eating times, walk timetables, recess, and sleep time. This consistency resembles pup Xanax - it chills them out.

- **Regard the Limits, Fella:** Read your canine's non-verbal communication. Try not to compel them to wear that charming vegetarian fleece sweater assuming they're giving you significant side-eye.

- **Persistence is an Ethicalness (Particularly While Managing Fastidious Eaters):** Changing to a without meat diet or changing in accordance with another home could take some time. Show restraint, understanding, and recollect, a cheerful vegetarian doggo is a slobber commendable doggo. Building Areas of strength for a: Indeed, you could simply throw a few kibble and tap out, yet for the insightful veggie lover doggo, a more edified approach is required. This is the way to make a harmony doggie lair that will cause your little guy to feel like the Dalai Lama of flavorful plant-based feasts: Uplifting feedback (since treats are the way in to any canine's heart, even a tofu-cherishing one): Trench the miserable, saturated milk-bones and investigate the universe of connoisseur veggie lover canine treats! Think dried out yam cuts, lentil emblems, or even - wheeze! - kale chips (simply joking... most likely). Use these morsels of plant-powered goodness to bribe, I mean, train your dog into the most obedient, well-behaved pup this side of the Himalayas.

- **Family Feud - Vegan Dog Edition:** If you share your abode with a pack of humans, make sure they're all on board with the vegan doggo lifestyle. Nobody wants a rogue uncle sneaking your pup a juicy steak behind your back (unless it's a vegan steak, then by all means, uncle!).

- **The Zen Vet Whisperer:** Got questions about your vegan dog's emotional well-being? Don't fret! Consult your friendly neighborhood vet. They'll be happy to answer your burning questions like, "Is it normal for Fido to meditate for hours on end?" (Spoiler alert: probably not, but they can still help!). Remember that creating a loving environment doesn't happen overnight (unless you're a master dog whisperer, in which case congratulations). Building a bond takes time and a lot of scribbles. Shower your vegetarian little guy with adoration, consideration, and those very significant gut rubs. The more grounded your bond, the more joyful your little guy (and the more uncertain they are to organize a tofu-based resistance). By following these tips, you'll transform your home into a haven for your plant-powered pup, and who knows, maybe you'll even pick up some mindfulness practices along the way (namaste, fellow dog lover!).

The End

Dear reader,

I extend my heartfelt gratitude for acquiring a copy of this work. Your decision to embrace it fills me with immense joy, knowing that I have been able to offer assistance through my words.

In the spirit of sharing joy, I kindly request you to consider leaving a review and spreading the word among others. Your support holds significant meaning to me.

If, by any chance, this piece did not meet your expectations, please accept my sincere apologies.

I assure you that I am committed to improving and striving for excellence in future endeavors. However, above all else, please remember that your act of acquiring this copy demonstrates that you are cherished and loved.

Once again, thank you for your support and for being a part of this journey.

Warm regards,

[Richard L. Dean]

RICHARD L . DEAN